Study Guide

for use with

Abnormal Psychology

Fourth Edition

Susan Nolen-Hoeksema

Prepared by

Jennifer Boothby
Indiana State University

Mc Graw Hill

Boston   Burr Ridge, IL   Dubuque, IA   Madison, WI   New York   San Francisco   St. Louis
Bangkok   Bogotá   Caracas   Kuala Lumpur   Lisbon   London   Madrid   Mexico City
Milan   Montreal   New Delhi   Santiago   Seoul   Singapore   Sydney   Taipei   Toronto

The McGraw·Hill Companies

McGraw-Hill Higher Education

Study Guide for use with
Abnormal Psychology
Susan Nolen-Hoeksema

Published by McGraw-Hill, an imprint of The McGraw-Hill Companies, Inc., 1221 Avenue of the Americas, New York, NY 10020. Copyright © 2007, 2004 by The McGraw-Hill Companies, Inc. All rights reserved. No part of this publication may be reproduced or distributed in any form or by any means, or stored in a database or retrieval system, without the prior written consent of The McGraw-Hill Companies, Inc., including, but not limited to, in any network or other electronic storage or transmission, or broadcast for distance learning.

1 2 3 4 5 6 7 8 9 0 QPD/QPD 0 9 8 7 6 5

ISBN-13: 978-0-07-319142-3
ISBN-10:   0-07-319142-6

www.mhhe.com

CONTENTS

Chapter 1: Looking at Abnormality

LEARNING OBJECTIVES

After reading and studying this chapter, you should be able to:

1. Discuss the factors that influence whether a behavior is regarded as normal or abnormal.

2. Summarize the different criteria for defining abnormality, and know the strengths and weaknesses of each criterion.

3. Describe the components of maladaptive behavior and how culture and gender may influence maladaptive behavior.

4. Distinguish among supernatural, biological, and psychological theories of abnormality, and discuss how each type of theory has led to different ways of treating mentally ill people throughout history.

5. Summarize how people from the Stone Age, the ancient Chinese, Egyptians, Greeks, and Hebrews thought about abnormality, and how each respective culture treated the mentally ill as a result.

6. Discuss the historical shift from the early asylums in Europe and America to the moral treatment movement.

7. Identify some of the notable figures in psychology from the late 19th and early-to-mid 20th centuries.

8. Discuss the goal of the deinstitutionalization movement, how communities attempted to achieve that goal, and whether such efforts were successful.

9. Discuss the advantages and disadvantages of managed care systems of mental health care service delivery.

10. Discuss the professions within abnormal psychology and how they differ from one another.

ESSENTIAL IDEAS

I. Defining abnormality

    A. Cultural relativism is a perspective on abnormality that argues that the norms of a society must be used to determine the normality of a behavior.

    B. The unusualness criterion for abnormality suggests that unusual or rare behaviors should be labeled abnormal.

C. The discomfort criterion suggests that only behaviors or emotions that an individual finds distressing should be labeled abnormal.

D. The mental illness criterion for abnormality suggests that only behaviors resulting from mental illness or disease are abnormal.

E. The consensus among professionals in the mental health field is that behaviors that cause people to suffer distress, that prevent them from functioning in daily life, and that are unusual are abnormal. Often these behaviors are referred to as *maladaptive*, and can be remembered by the 3Ds: distress, dysfunction, and deviance.

II. Historical perspectives on abnormality

A. Three types of theories have influenced the definition and treatment of abnormality over the ages: the biological theories, the supernatural theories, and the psychological theories.

B. Stone Age people probably viewed abnormal behavior as a result of supernatural forces. They may have drilled holes in the skulls of sufferers – a procedure known as trephination – to release the evil forces causing the abnormal behavior.

C. Some of the earliest written references to abnormal behavior can be found in Chinese medical texts around 2674 B.C.; in the papyri of Egypt and Mesopotamia; in the Old Testament; and in the writings of Greek and Roman philosophers and physicians. Abnormal behaviors were often described as medical disorders in these ancient writings, although there is also evidence that they were attributed to supernatural forces.

D. The witch hunts began in the late Middle Ages. Some accused witches may have suffered from abnormal behavior.

E. Psychic epidemics have occurred throughout history. They were once attributed to spirit possession but are now attributed to the effects of social conditions on people's self-perceptions.

F. In the 18th and 19th centuries, advocates of more gentle treatment of people with abnormal behavior began to establish asylums for these people.

III. The emergence of modern perspectives

A. Modern biological theories and therapies began with the development of Kraepelin's classification scheme for psychological disorders and the discovery that syphillis causes general paresis, a disease with symptoms that include losing touch with reality.

B. The roots of psychoanalytic theory can be found in the work of Mesmer and the suggestion that psychological symptoms can be relieved through hypnosis. Jean Charcot,

Sigmund Freud, and Josef Breuer are among the founders of modern psychoanalytic theory, which focuses on the role of the unconscious in psychological symptoms.

C. Behavioral approaches to psychopathology began with the development of basic experimental techniques to study the effects of reinforcements and punishments in producing normal and abnormal behavior.

D. Cognitive approaches to abnormality emerged in the mid-20th century, when theorists began arguing that the way people think about events in their environment determines their emotional and behavioral responses to those events.

IV. Modern mental health care

A. The goal of the deinstitutionalization movement was to move mental patients from custodial mental health facilities, where they were isolated and received little treatment, to community-based mental health centers. Thousands of patients were released from mental institutions. Unfortunately, community-based mental health centers have never been fully funded or supported, leaving many former mental patients with few resources in the community.

B. Managed care systems are meant to provide coordinated, comprehensive medical care to patients. This can be a great asset to people with long-term, serious mental disorders. Coverage for mental health problems tends to be limited, however, and many people have no insurance at all.

C. A number of professions provide care to people with mental health problems, including psychiatrists, psychologists, marriage and family therapists, clinical social workers, and psychiatric nurses.

KEY TERMS AND GUIDED REVIEW

Key Terms

psychopathology:

Defining Abnormality

Key Terms

context:

cultural relativism:

gender roles:

unusualness:

discomfort:

mental illness:

maladaptive:

<u>Guided Review</u>

1. Give an example of a behavior that would be considered abnormal in one context, but not in another context.

2. Give some examples of how culture and gender can affect the expression and experience of maladaptive behaviors.

3. What is Thomas Szasz's view of cultural relativism?

4. What are some advantages and disadvantages of adopting the cultural relativism criterion for abnormality?

5. How are the cultural relativism criterion and the unusualness criterion similar?

6. Give one advantage and one disadvantage of adopting the unusualness criterion as a standard for defining abnormal behavior.

7. Give one advantage and one disadvantage of adopting the discomfort criterion as a standard for defining abnormal behavior.

8. What is one problem with the mental illness criterion?

9. What are the three components of the maladaptiveness criterion?

Historical Perspectives on Abnormality

<u>Key Terms</u>

biological theories:

supernatural theories:

psychological theories:

trephination:

psychic epidemic:

moral treatment:

1. During the Stone Age, what was thought to cause abnormal behavior, and what was the prescribed treatment?

2. Summarize the concepts of "yin and yang" and "vital air" from ancient China.

3. What did the Egyptians and Greeks believe was responsible for psychological problems? How did they attempt to treat these problems?

4. What was the Hebrews' conception of abnormal behavior (as depicted in the Old Testament), and how did they believe abnormal behavior should be treated?

5. How did Hipprocates and Plato view abnormal behavior? How did their views differ?

6. During ancient times, how were people with abnormal behavior treated by society?

7. Describe the shift that occurred during the Middle Ages in which the causes of abnormal behavior came to be viewed differently.

8. Why might some people have actually believed they were witches?

9. What was Saint Vitus' dance? What was tarantism?

10. Describe how people with abnormal behavior were treated during the eighteenth and nineteenth centuries in Europe and America.

11. How did Dorothea Dix and Philippe Pinel contribute to the treatment of people with abnormal behavior?

12. What led to the decline of the moral treatment movement?

The Emergence of Modern Perspectives

Key Terms

general paresis:

mesmerism:

psychoanalysis:

behaviorism:

cognitions:

self-efficacy beliefs:

<u>Guided Review</u>

1. What was Emil Kraepelin's contribution to our understanding of mental disorders?

2. Describe one event that increased acceptance of biological explanations of abnormality.

3. According to Mesmer, what caused psychological disorders and how could they be treated? How did Mesmer contribute to the development of psychoanalysis?

4. What persuaded Charcot to believe that hysteria had psychological roots?

5. How did Breuer contribute to the development of psychoanalysis?

6. Summarize the contributions of Wundt, Witmer, Pavlov, Watson, Thorndike, and Skinner to the development of behaviorism.

7. Summarize the contributions of Bandura, Ellis, and Beck to the study of cognitive views of abnormality.

8. How do supernatural theories continue to affect the practice of psychotherapy?

Modern Mental Health Care

<u>Key Terms</u>

patients' rights movement:

deinstitutionalization:

community mental health movement:

managed care:

<u>Guided Review</u>

1. What were some advantages and disadvantages of the patients' rights and community mental health movements?

2. What are some advantages and disadvantages of managed health care?

Professions within Abnormal Psychology

Guided Review

1. How are psychiatrists, clinical psychologists, marriage and family therapists, clinical social workers, and psychiatric nurses similar and different?

Chapter Integration

Key Terms

integrationist approach:

mental hygiene movement:

Guided Review

1. Who was Clifford Beers, what happened to him, and how did he affect the public's view of abnormal behavior?

CHAPTER TEST

A. Multiple Choice. Choose the **best answer** to each question below.

1. People must suffer as a result of their behavior according to the _____, but not necessarily according to the _____.

    A. maladaptiveness criterion; cultural relativism criterion.
    B. mental illness criterion; discomfort criterion.
    C. cultural relativism criterion; unusualness criterion.
    D. discomfort criterion; unusualness criterion.

2. One problem with accepting the cultural relativism criterion is

    A. cultures may differ in how they define abnormal behavior.
    B. some societies may label people or groups abnormal in order to justify controlling them.
    C. some groups, such as gay men and lesbians, do not find their behavior distressing.
    D. someone still has to decide how rare a behavior must be for it to be called abnormal.

3. The _____ criterion was responsible for _____.

    A. maladaptiveness; the imprisonment of Thomas Szasz.
    B. unusualness; the removal of homosexuality from the APA list of recognized psychological disorders.
    C. mental illness; the labeling of slaves who desired freedom as having drapetomania.

D. discomfort; the removal of homosexuality from the APA list of recognized psychological disorders.

4. All of the following are components of the maladaptiveness criterion except:

    A. the behaviors occur for only brief periods of time.
    B. the behaviors are highly unusual.
    C. the behaviors result in psychological discomfort.
    D. the behaviors interfere with the person's ability to function in daily life.

5. The idea that the flowing of "vital air" on specific body organs controls emotions was a _____ theory and was developed by the _____

    A. supernatural; Hebrews
    B. psychological; Greeks
    C. supernatural; Egyptians
    D. biological; Chinese

6. The _____ believed that a "wandering uterus" traveled around the female body, interfered with other organs, and caused _____.

    A. Chinese; hysteria
    B. Europeans; witchcraft and obscene behavior
    C. Greeks and Egyptians; hysteria
    D. Hebrews; melancholia

7. Which of the following is true about a culture and its discovery?

    A. The Egyptians assigned mental functioning to the brain.
    B. The Greeks first drew the distinction between madness and witchcraft.
    C. The Chinese developed the first effective "talk" therapies for mental disorders.
    D. The Hebrews developed the first true systematic classification system of mental disorders.

8. The Hebrews believed that abnormal behavior could be treated through

    A. ritual dancing.
    B. achieving a balance of bodily fluids.
    C. smelling substances with strong odors.
    D. the confession of sins.

9. Greek physicians believed that _____ caused psychological problems, and that the best type of treatment would involve _____.

    A. an imbalance of four humors (blood, phlegm, yellow bile, and black bile); physiological alterations or psychological treatments such as rest, relaxation, or

change of lifestyle.
B. afflictions from the gods; trephination.
C. vital air blowing on specific body organs; restoration of the body to a more balanced state by rest, relaxation, and herbal medicine.
D. moral vice and sloth; a life of reason, rationality, and virtue.

10. Which of the following writings argued that many people accused of witchcraft actually suffered from mental illness?

    A. <u>A Mind that Found Itself</u>
    B. <u>The Deception of Dreams</u>
    C. <u>Papyrus Ebers</u>
    D. <u>The Old Testament</u>

11. What tends to characterize psychic epidemics and mass hysteria is

    A. the fact that they can only occur in superstitious cultures.
    B. the fact that the participants are trying to express their emotions, yet lack an adaptive way to do this, and thus participate in psychic epidemics.
    C. the fact that they begin with one person, who then incites others to imitate the same behavioral symptoms.
    D. the fact that the participants suffer from psychological distress rather than an identifiable physical illness.

12. Which of the following people was associated with the moral treatment movement, and which statement best characterizes the beliefs of the movement?

    A. Clifford Beers; mental disorders result from blasphemy and the abandonment of religion: the purpose of treatment is to restore people's morality so that they might function again.
    B. Teresa of Avila; mental disorders result from natural causes and should be treated biologically.
    C. Dorothea Dix; mental illness resulted from the separation of people from nature and stresses resulting from rapid social changes.
    D. Philippe Pinel; hospitals should isolate mentally ill people to keep their immorality from afflicting the general populace.

13. All of the following contributed to the demise of the moral treatment movement toward the end of the nineteenth century except:

    A. Many patients failed to improve or got worse.
    B. The expansion of asylums created a shortage of personnel and resources.
    C. Biological treatments were developed and were more effective.
    D. An increasing number of asylum patients were from foreign countries.

14. Which individual is known for developing a classification scheme for mental disorders?

A. Jean Charcot
B. Emil Kraepelin
C. Aaron Beck
D. E. L. Thorndike

15. A significant event that increased awareness that mental illness can have biological causes was

A. the publication of <u>On the Psychical Mechanisms of Hysterical Phenomena.</u>
B. the discovery that untreated streptococcus can cause schizophrenia.
C. the laboratory experiments of Kraepelin.
D. the discovery that syphilis could cause general paresis.

16. _____ classified mental disorders into epilepsy, mania, melancholia, and brain fever.

A. Kraepelin
B. Hippocrates
C. Freud
D. Charcot

17. _____ is a technique used in _____.

A. Mesmerism; classical conditioning
B. Trephination; hypnosis
C. Hypnosis; mesmerism
D. Classical conditioning; psychoanalysis

18. _____ developed _____, which greatly influenced modern thinking.

A. Anton Mesmer; psychoanalysis
B. Emil Kraepelin; a classification system for mental disorders
C. Willhelm Wundt; hypnosis
D. Joseph Breuer; the first experimental psychology laboratory

19. Which of the following was instrumental in showing that behaviors followed by positive consequences were more likely to be repeated than behaviors followed by negative consequences?

A. B.F. Skinner
B. Ivan Pavlov
C. Albert Ellis
D. Lightner Witmer

20. When helping someone with a psychological disorder, which of the following professionals would be most likely to focus on overcoming environmental conditions contributing to the person's problems, such as homelessness?

     A. Psychiatrists
     B. Psychiatric nurses
     C. Social workers
     D. Clinical psychologists

B. <u>True-False</u>. Select T (True) or F (False) below.

1. Supernatural theories no longer have any influence on the treatment of people with mental disorders by clinical psychologists.　T　　F

2. In the early 1970s, homosexual men and women were found to experience more psychological distress than heterosexuals, and the diagnosis of homosexuality was removed in order to encourage a focus on the psychological problems of homosexuals, rather than the diagnosis itself.　T　　F

3. People who do not consider their own behavior to be abnormal cannot be considered abnormal according to cultural relativism.　　T　　F

4. Culture and gender influence how likely it is that a given maladaptive behavior will be shown, as well as people's willingness to admit to certain kinds of maladaptive behaviors.
    T　　F

5. Biological views have invariably led to more compassion for people afflicted with mental illness.　　T　　F

C. <u>Short Answer Questions.</u>

1. List three criteria for defining abnormality. For each criterion, provide one argument in favor of the criterion and one argument against it.

2. Briefly discuss how "change came from within" to alter many people's views of those accused of being witches in the 16th century.

3. Give two historical examples of how a particular view of the cause(s) of abnormal behavior influenced views of the most appropriate treatment for the behavior.

4. What 19th century event provided strong evidence that some abnormal behavior has biological causes? Describe this event.

5. Briefly discuss the impact of health insurance on the treatment of mental health problems.

ANSWER KEY

Multiple Choice
1. D
2. B
3. D
4. A
5. D
6. C
7. A
8. D
9. A
10. B
11. D
12. C
13. C
14. B
15. D
16. B
17. C
18. B
19. A
20. C

True-False
1. F
2. F
3. F
4. T
5. F

Short Answer Questions
1. See pp. 5-11.
2. See p. 16.
3. See p. 10-21.
4. See pp. 21-22.
5. See pp. 24-26.

Additional Readings on Chapter 1 Topics
Greenwood, J. D. (1999). Understanding the "cognitive revolution" in psychology. Journal of the History of the Behavioral Sciences, 35, 1-22.
Kraepelin, E. (1992). The manifestations of insanity. History of Psychiatry, 3, 509-529.
Wilson, K. (1997). Science and treatment development: Lessons from the history of behavior therapy. Behavior Therapy, 28, 547-558.

Chapter 2: Contemporary Theories of Abnormality

LEARNING OBJECTIVES

After reading and studying this chapter, you should be able to:

1. Distinguish among biological, psychological, and social approaches to abnormality, and discuss how each approach leads to different conceptions of the causes of abnormality. Also, discuss how these approaches are not mutually exclusive, and summarize how advocates of all approaches might work together to develop integrated models for understanding abnormality.

2. Discuss the three biological causes of abnormality, and describe the relationship between structural brain abnormalities and psychological impairment. Summarize the processes involved in communication between neurons, and what aspects of this process may break down, resulting in psychological distress. Summarize how researchers investigate genetic contributions to psychopathology, and the current polygenic model.

3. Describe the basic foundation of psychodynamic theory, and know each defense mechanism. Discuss how Erikson and the object relations school differ from the traditional psychodynamic perspective.

4. Summarize classical and operant conditioning, and give examples of each.

5. Discuss Bandura's social learning theory, and relate it to both the "pure" behavioral theories and the cognitive theories.

6. Know and be able to distinguish among causal attributions, control beliefs, self-efficacy, and global assumptions.

7. Discuss the elements of both humanistic and existential theories, and describe how they differ.

8. Discuss the social theories of abnormality in terms of the hypothesized role of interpersonal relationships, family dynamics, and the larger society in producing psychological symptoms.

ESSENTIAL IDEAS

I. Biological approaches

    A. The biological theories of psychopathology hold that psychological symptoms and disorders are caused by structural abnormalities in the brain, disordered biochemistry, or faulty genes.

    B. Structural abnormalities in the brain can be caused by injury or disease processes. The location of brain damage influences the type of psychological symptoms shown.

C. Most biochemical theories focus on neurotransmitters, the substances that facilitate the transmission of impulses in the brain. Some theories say that psychological symptoms are caused by too little or too much of a particular neurotransmitter in the synapses of the brain. Other theories focus on the number of receptors for neurotransmitters.

D. Some people may be genetically predisposed to psychological disorders. Most of these disorders are probably linked not to a single faulty gene but to the accumulation of a group of faulty genes.

E. Three methods of determining the heritability of a disorder are family history studies, twin studies, and adoption studies.

II. Psychological approaches

A. Psychodynamic theories of psychopathology focus on unconscious conflicts that cause anxiety and result in maladaptive behavior.

B. The ways people handle their conflicts are defined by the types of defense mechanisms they use. Children can become fixated on certain needs or concerns if their transitions through psychosexual stages are not managed well.

C. More recent psychodynamic theories focus less on the role of unconscious impulses and more on the development of the individual's self-concept in the context of interpersonal relationships. They see a greater role for the environment in the shaping of personality and have more hope for change in personality during adulthood than Freud did.

D. The behavioral theories of abnormality focus only on the rewards and punishments in the environment that shape and maintain behavior.

E. Classical conditioning takes place when a previously neutral stimulus is paired with a stimulus that naturally creates a certain response. Eventually the neutral stimulus will also elicit the response.

F. Operant conditioning involves rewarding desired behaviors and punishing undesired behaviors.

G. People also learn by imitating the behaviors modeled by others and by observing the rewards and punishments others receive for their behaviors.

H. Cognitive theories suggest that people's attributions for events, their perceptions of control and self-efficacy, and their global assumptions about themselves and the world influence their behaviors and emotions in reaction to situations.

I. Humanist and existential theories suggest that all humans strive to fulfill their potential for good and to self-actualize. The inability to fulfill one's potential arises from the pressures of society to conform to others' expectations and values and from existential anxiety.

III. Social and Interpersonal approaches

A. The interpersonal theories assert that our self-concepts and expectations of others are based on our early attachments and relationships to caregivers.

B. Family systems theories suggest that families form cohesive systems, which regulate the behavior of each member in the system. Sometimes these systems support and enhance the well-being of their members but sometimes they do not.

C. Social structural theories suggest that society contributes to psychopathology in some people by creating severe stresses for them, then allowing or encouraging them to cope with these stresses with psychological symptoms. People living in chronically stressful environments have higher rates of psychopathology.

KEY TERMS AND GUIDED REVIEW

<u>Key Terms</u>

theory:

biological approach:

psychological approach:

social approach:

vulnerability-stress models:

<u>Guided Review</u>

1. Give an example of how biological, psychological, and social factors can combine with stress to cause a disorder.

Biological Approaches

<u>Key Terms</u>

cerebral cortex:

hypothalamus:

limbic system:

neurotransmitters:

synapse:

receptors:

reuptake:

degradation:

endocrine system:

hormone:

pituitary:

behavior genetics:

polygenic:

predisposition:

family history study:

monozygotic (MZ) twins:

dizygotic (DZ) twins:

twin study:

concordance rate:

adoption study:

Guided Review

1. What are the functions of the hypothalamus? What role does the limbic system play with respect to the hypothalamus?

2. Summarize the steps involved in the process of neurotransmission, or communication between neurons.

3. What two natural processes govern the regulation of neurotransmitters in the synapse? What happens when these processes are disrupted?

4. Name two neurotransmitters and describe how they potentially affect psychological functioning.

5. Describe the components of the HPA axis and the sequence of chemical events during a stress response.

6. How are chromosomes, genes, and DNA related?

7. How is a family history study conducted? What is a major limitation of family history studies?

8. Write the expected concordance rates for the following scenarios: a) a disorder is determined entirely by genetics; b) a disorder is determined partly by genetics; c) a disorder is not determined by genetics at all.

a. MZ = _____   DZ = _____
b. MZ = _____   DZ = _____
c. MZ = _____   DZ = _____

9. What is one limitation of twin studies?

10. How is an adoption study conducted? What is one limitation of these studies?

11. What are some of the limitations of biological theories? Why does it seem that the general public has embraced them?

Psychological Approaches

Key Terms

psychodynamic theories:

psychoanalysis:

catharsis:

repression:

libido:

id:

pleasure principle:

primary process thinking:

ego:

reality principle:

secondary process thinking:

superego:

introject:

unconscious:

preconscious:

conscious:

defense mechanism:

neurotic paradox:

psychosexual stages:

oral stage:

anal stage:

phallic stage:

Oedipus complex:

castration anxiety:

Electra complex:

penis envy:

latency stage:

genital stage:

object relations:

splitting:

behavioral theories:

classical conditioning:

unconditioned stimulus (US):

unconditioned response (UR):

conditioned stimulus (CS):

conditioned response (CR):

operant conditioning:

continuous reinforcement schedule:

partial reinforcement schedule:

extinction:

social learning theory:

modeling:

observational learning:

cognitive theories:

cognitions:

causal attribution:

control theory:

global assumptions:

humanistic theories:

existential theories:

self-actualization:

client-centered therapy:

<u>Guided Review</u>

1. What early observations influenced Freud's thinking and the development of psychoanalysis?

2. From the perspective of psychodynamic theory, describe how the id, ego, and superego would interact given the following situation:

> A hungry young child sees an open cookie jar on the counter. His mother told him a few minutes ago not to have any snacks before dinner. He stares longingly at the cookie jar, but remembers what his mother has just told him.

What impulse or need would each component of the psyche attempt to satisfy, and within what principles would each operate in this example?

3. How does the ego prevent threatening material from reaching the conscious mind?

4. What are Freud's five stages of psychosexual development? Describe each stage, and indicate what personality characteristics are thought to develop if each stage is not completed properly.

5. How do boys and girls develop a value system, according to Freud?

6. According to object relations theory, what are the four steps in the development of a self-concept?

7. What are some of the limitations of Freudian theory?

8. A woman who is chewing gum stumbles upon a large snake, which startles her. She screams and runs away from the snake. A week later, when a friend offers her a piece of gum, she screams and runs away from her friend. Identify the unconditioned stimulus, unconditioned response, conditioned stimulus, and conditioned response in this story.

9. How do continuous reinforcement schedules and partial reinforcement schedules differ, and how do these schedules impact the process of extinction?

10. According to social learning theory, what are two mechanisms of learning? Explain how Bandura's social learning theory and Freud's theory of defense mechanisms would each explain the behavior of a prisoner who began to act like the guards at his or her prison.

11. What are some strengths and weaknesses of behavioral theories?

12. Give an example of how causal attributions can affect one's emotional responses to situations.

13. Explain what self-efficacy is, and give an example of how a sense of self-efficacy might impact an individual's response to a stressful situation.

14. Give some examples of dysfunctional assumptions.

15. What are some strengths and weaknesses of cognitive theories?

16. According to humanistic theories, what might lead individuals to feel distress?

17. What are some strengths and weaknesses of humanistic/existential theories?

Social and Interpersonal Approaches

Key Terms

interpersonal theories:

prototypes:

family systems theories:

social structural theories:

Guided Review

1. How do the theories of Adler and Erikson differ from Freud's theory?

2. Describe Sullivan's (1953) theory. How does it differ from object relations theory and operant conditioning?

3. What is Bowlby's (1980) theory, and how might it explain abnormal behavior in adults?

4. According to family systems theory, how might the family environment contribute to psychopathology? Give an example.

5. Describe some societal factors that might contribute to abnormal behavior in individuals.

6. What are some strengths and weaknesses of social and interpersonal theories?

CHAPTER TEST

A. <u>Multiple Choice.</u> Choose the **best answer** to each question below.

1. Albert Ellis attributed his fear of public speaking to

    A. irrational beliefs.
    B. past experiences of rejection.
    C. a genetic predisposition to anxiety.
    D. a dysfunction in his GABA system.

2. The _____ releases _____, which causes the _____ to release adrenocorticotrophic hormone.

    A. pituitary; growth hormone; hypothalamus
    B. hypothalamus; corticotrophin-releasing factor; pituitary
    C. pituitary; corticotrophin-releasing factor; adrenal gland
    D. cerebrum; serotonin; adrenal gland

3. Choose the correct order of the following steps involved in communication between neurons: 1) neurotransmitters bind to the dendrites of the receiving neuron; 2) a signal travels through the axon of the sending neuron; 3) neurotransmitter is released into the synapse; 4) the receiving neuron is stimulated to initiate an impulse; 5) the signal reaches the synaptic terminals of the sending neuron.

    A. 5, 2, 1, 3, 4
    B. 3, 2, 5, 4, 1

C. 2, 3, 1, 5, 4
D. 2, 5, 3, 1, 4

4. Inhibiting the process of reuptake in a neuron leads to

   A. Compensation by means of increasing the frequency of degradation.
   B. A greater amount of neurotransmitter in the synapse.
   C. A lesser amount of neurotransmitter in the synapse.
   D. An increase in the number of dendrite receptors on the receiving neuron.

5. Judy has an anxiety disorder, but no one in her immediate family has ever had one, nor has any of her past relatives. How is this possible, according to what the chapter discussed about genetic transmission of mental disorders?

   A. Judy must have been adopted.
   B. Judy may have received enough abnormal genes from the chromosomes of her mother and father at birth to inevitably cause an anxiety disorder.
   C. Some of Judy's family members may actually carry a predisposition for an anxiety disorder, but may never have experienced an interaction among genetic, biological, and environmental factors sufficient to cause the disorder.
   D. The situation described is not possible according to what we know about genetics.

6. Investigators at the University of Planet Earth wanted to understand the biological roots of moon disorder, a condition in which individuals experience symptoms of depression and anxiety because they cannot live on the moon. They found a large sample of people who had moon disorder, and a large sample of people who did not have moon disorder. After analyzing the genetic history of these two groups, they found that significantly more relatives of the moon disorder group also had moon disorder, compared to the relatives of the group without moon disorder. Next, they examined the concordance rate of moon disorder among both monozygotic and dizygotic twins in the sample. The concordance rate of moon disorder was 43 percent among MZ twins, and was the same among DZ twins. What can the investigators conclude?

   A. There is substantial evidence that moon disorder is genetically transmitted.
   B. There is some evidence that moon disorder is genetically transmitted, but an adoption study would be necessary to tease apart genetic from environmental factors.
   C. There is no evidence that moon disorder is genetically transmitted, but there is some evidence that moon disorder occurs among people who share similar environments.
   D. There is no evidence that the rate of moon disorder is influenced either by genetic or environmental factors.

7. Leroy has just come home from a bad day at work. His boss ridiculed him at a group meeting because he did not have a report that had been due a week earlier. His dog comes running up to him, carrying his food dish in his mouth, wagging its tail excitedly. "You stupid mutt," he exclaims angrily, "you're always trying to torment me and remind me of what I forgot to do!" This is most likely an illustration of which defense mechanism?

A. Reaction formation
B. Rationalization
C. Projection
D. Displacement

8. According to Freud, _____ is responsible for _____.

    A. castration anxiety; penis envy
    B. the superego; channeling libido into activities that balance the demands of society and the moral conscience
    C. introjection; incorporation of the standards of others into one's own thinking
    D. the preconscious; the release of emotions connected to memories and conflicts.

9. A woman who is hungry for lunch, but who is stuck in a meeting until 1:30 P.M. and manages to avoid eating, is engaging in _____ which is controlled by the _____.

    A. primary process thinking; superego
    B. secondary process thinking; ego
    C. introjection; preconscious
    D. the reality principle; superego

10. The _____ stage lasts from _____, and if not resolved properly, an individual can be _____ as an adult.

    A. oral; 18 months to 3 years of age; stubborn, overcontrolling, and focused on orderliness
    B. anal; 6 years of age to puberty; have a deep mistrust of others and fear of abandonment
    C. phallic; 3 to 6 years of age; too self-aggrandizing or too self-deprecating
    D. latency; 3 to 6 years of age; riddled with hatred of the opposite sex

11. According to object relations theory, in which of the following phases of self-concept development does the child see the self as either all-good or all-bad and others as either all-good or all-bad, and is able to distinguish between the self and others?

    A. Separation-individuation
    B. Symbiosis
    C. Integration
    D. Undifferentiated

12. Which of the following is not one of Horney's criticisms of psychodynamic theory?

    A. Psychodynamic theory views males as prototypical human beings.
    B. Psychodynamic theory wrongly attempts to explain normal and abnormal behavior with similar processes.
    C. Psychodynamic theory overemphasizes sexual drives and anatomy in personality.

D. Psychodynamic theory attempts to explain all human behavior based on a small sample.

13. Bill is running outside in his white tennis shoes when he looks down to see a snake slithering near his feet. Terrified, he yelps and half runs/half dances to get around the snake. The next morning, Bill experiences fear and anxiety when he starts to put on his shoes. The shoes are the

    A. unconditioned stimulus.
    B. conditioned response.
    C. unconditioned response.
    D. conditioned stimulus.

14. To shape and maintain a behavior, the most efficient means would be _____, but if a behavior were learned by means of _____, then it would be _____ to extinguish.

    A. classical conditioning; operant conditioning; more difficult
    B. operant conditioning; classical conditioning; less difficult
    C. a continuous reinforcement schedule; a partial reinforcement schedule; more difficult
    D. a continuous reinforcement schedule; a partial reinforcement schedule; less difficult

15. A major problem for cognitive theories is

    A. the fact that they are abstract and cannot be tested scientifically.
    B. the fact that they do not seem to recognize people's "free will."
    C. the fact that they have not shown convincingly that cognitions precede and cause disorders.
    D. the fact that they are studied in laboratories that do not resemble the real world.

16. Categorize the thought processes in the individual described below:

    Maria is very upset because she was supposed to start taking tennis lessons with her best friend Jane. Jane, however, decided to take lessons in another league that was closer to her home. (i) "Jane is so selfish," thought Maria, "and always thinks only of her own needs."
    Maria started taking the tennis lessons anyway, but became very dismayed when she learned how much physical work was involved. (ii) "I should be able to do this with absolute perfection! It looks so simple and graceful when I watch other people; I should be able to do this correctly just like they do!"

    A. (i) causal attribution; (ii) dysfunctional assumption
    B. (i) dysfunctional assumption; (ii) control belief
    C. (i). control belief; (ii) self-efficacy expectation
    D. (i) dysfunctional assumption; (ii) learned helplessness

17. According to Maslow, needs for security and an absence of danger are called _____

and must be met after _____ needs.

        A. belongingness and love needs; aesthetic
        B. esteem needs; self-actualization
        C. safety needs; physiological
        D. physiological; cognitive

18. According to Erikson, individuals pass through a psychosocial crisis known as _____ when they are in early adulthood.

        A. identity vs. confusion
        B. integrity vs. despair
        C. initiative vs. guilt
        D. intimacy vs. isolation

19. The family system seeks to maintain _____, according to family systems theorists.

        A. strong attachments
        B. homeostasis
        C. adaptive scripts
        D. triangular relationships

20. Proponents of social structural theories argue that abnormal behavior might develop from

        A. living in poverty-stricken neighborhoods.
        B. anxiety about our ultimate death.
        C. the structure of our dysfunctional assumptions.
        D. an inability to resolve psychosocial crises in relationships.

B. <u>True-False.</u> Select T (True) or F (False) below.

1. Phineas Gage became more quiet and responsible following his brain injury.
      T   F

2. Neither family history studies nor twin studies can tease apart the influence of genes versus the environment in shaping personality.   T   F

3. Castration anxiety is responsible for resolution of the Oedipus complex in boys.
      T   F

4. According to object relations theory, symbiosis is the stage at which the infant cannot distinguish between self and other, but does distinguish between good and bad aspects of the self-plus-other image.   T   F

5. B.F. Skinner's main contribution to psychology was the description and validation of observational learning as a learning mechanism.   T   F

C. <u>Short Answer Questions.</u>

1. Define behavior genetics and briefly describe the possible role of genetics in the development of psychological disorders.

2. Describe the three types of studies used to test genetic hypotheses of mental disorders. What is one limitation of each method?

3. Summarize Freud's five stages of psychosexual development.

4. What are some advantages and disadvantages of psychodynamic theory?

5. Summarize Bowlby's theory of normal and abnormal behavior.

ANSWER KEY

<u>Multiple Choice</u>
1. A
2. B
3. D
4. B
5. C
6. C
7. D
8. C
9. B
10. C
11. A
12. B
13. D
14. C
15. C
16. A
17. C
18. D
19. B
20. A

<u>True-False</u>
1. F
2. T
3. T
4. T
5. F

<u>Short Answer Questions</u>
1. See pp. 42 -46.
2. See pp. 42-46.
3. See pp. 49-51.
4. See p. 53.
5. See p. 62.

<u>Additional Readings on Chapter 2 Topics</u>
Bandura, A. (2000). Social cognitive theory: An agentic perspective. <u>Annual Review of Psychology, 52,</u> 1-26.
Fonagy, P., & Target, M. (2000). The place of psychodynamic theory in developmental psychology. <u>Developmental Psychopathology, 12,</u> 407-425.

Schore, A. N. (1997). A century after Freud's project: Is a rapprochement between psychoanalysis and neurobiology at hand? <u>Journal of the American Psychoanalytic Association, 45,</u> 807-840.

Chapter 3: The Research Endeavor

LEARNING OBJECTIVES

After reading and studying this chapter, you should be able to:

1. Explain the challenges inherent in researching abnormal behavior and approaches for overcoming many of these obstacles.

2. Define and distinguish between a primary hypothesis and a null hypothesis.

3. Define and distinguish between independent and dependent variables.

4. Explain the concept of operationalization.

5. Discuss the advantages and disadvantages of case studies.

6. Describe and distinguish among continuous variable, group comparison, cross-sectional, longitudinal, epidemiological, human laboratory, therapy outcome, single-case experimental, and animal studies, as well as the strengths and limitations of each type of study.

7. Explain why it is important to have a representative sample.

8. Discuss what third variables are and how they may be minimized or eliminated.

9. Explain why it can be important to match research participants on certain variables when comparing two groups.

10. Discuss what "significant differences" are between groups, and how significance is determined.

11. Define and distinguish between the prevalence and incidence of a psychological disorder.

12. Define and distinguish among control groups, placebo control groups, wait list control groups, and experimental groups, and explain the circumstances in which each would be appropriate and why (with regard to therapy outcome studies).

13. Define and distinguish between treatment efficacy and treatment effectiveness.

13. Discuss the ethical problems raised by human laboratory, therapy outcome, and animal studies and ways in which researchers attempt to avoid these problems.

14. Discuss the value of cross-cultural research and the challenges inherent in conducting such research.

15. Discuss the advantages and disadvantages of meta-analysis.

ESSENTIAL IDEAS

I. The scientific method

    A. The scientific method is a set of steps designed to obtain and evaluate information relevant to a problem in a systematic way.

    B. A hypothesis is a testable statement of what we expect to happen in a research study.

    C. A null hypothesis is the statement that the outcome of the study will contradict the primary hypothesis of the study. Usually, the null hypothesis says that the variables (such as stress and depression) are unrelated to one another.

    D. A variable is a factor that can vary within individuals or between individuals.

    E. A dependent variable is the factor we are trying to predict in a study.

    F. An independent variable is the factor we are using to predict the dependent variable.

    G. Operationalization is the way we measure or manipulate the variables of interest.

II. Case studies

    A. Case studies are in-depth histories of the experiences of individuals.

    B. The advantages of case studies are their richness in detail, their attention to the unique experiences of individuals, their ability to focus on rare problems, and their ability to generate new ideas.

    C. The disadvantages of case studies are their lack of generalizability, their lack of objectivity, and difficulties in replication.

III. Correlational studies

    A. A correlational study examines the relationship between two variables without manipulating either variable.

    B. A correlation coefficient is an index of the relationship between two variables. It can range from -1.00 to $+1.00$. The magnitude of the correlation indicates how strong the relationship between the variables is.

    C. A positive correlation indicates that, as values of one variable increase, values of the other variable increase. A negative correlation indicates that, as values of one variable increase, values of the other variable decrease.

D. A result is said to be statistically significant if it is unlikely to have happened by chance. The convention in psychological research is to accept results that have a probability of less than 5 in 100 of happening by chance.

E. A correlational study can show that two variables are related, but it cannot show that one variable causes the other.

F. All correlational studies suffer from the third variable problem—the possibility that variables not measured in the study actually account for the relationship between the variables measured in the study.

G. Continuous variable studies evaluate the relationship between two variables that vary along a continuum.

H. A sample is a subset of a population of interest. A representative sample is similar to the population on all important variables. One way to generate a representative sample is to obtain a random sample.

I. Cross-sectional studies assess a sample at one point in time, and longitudinal studies assess a sample at multiple points in time. A longitudinal study assesses a sample that is expected to have some key event in the future both before and after the event, then examines changes that occurred in the sample.

J. Group comparison studies evaluate differences between key groups, such as a group that experienced a specific type of stressor and a comparison group that did not experience the stressor but is matched on all important variables.

K. Potential problems in correlational studies include the potential for bad timing and the expense of longitudinal studies.

IV. Epidemiological studies

A. Epidemiology is the study of the frequency and distribution of a disorder in a population.

B. The prevalence of a disorder is the proportion of the population that has the disorder at a given point or period in time.

C. The incidence of a disorder is the number of new cases of the disorder that develop during a specific period of time.

D. Risk factors for a disorder are conditions or variables that are associated with a higher risk of having the disorder.

V. Experimental studies

A. Experimental studies attempt to control all variables affecting the dependent variable.

B. In human laboratory studies, the independent variable is manipulated and the effects on people participating in the study are examined. To control for the effects of being in the experimental situation and the passage of time, researchers use control groups, in which participants have all the same experiences as the group of main interest in the study, except that they do not receive the key manipulation.

C. Demand characteristics are aspects of the experimental situation that cause participants to guess the purpose of the study and change their behavior as a result.

D. Disadvantages of human laboratory studies include their lack of generalizability and the ethical issues involved in manipulating people.

E. Therapy outcome studies assess the impact of an intervention designed to relieve symptoms. Simple control groups, wait list control groups, and placebo control groups are used to compare the effects of the intervention with other alternatives.

F. It can be difficult to determine what aspects of a therapy resulted in changes in participants. Therapy outcome studies also can suffer from lack of generalizability, and assigning people who need treatment to control groups holds ethical implications.

G. Single-case experimental designs involve the intensive investigation of single individuals or small groups of individuals, before and after a manipulation or intervention.

H. In an ABAB or reversal design, an intervention is introduced, withdrawn, and then reinstated, and the behavior of a participant is examined on and off the treatment.

I. Animal studies involve exposing animals to conditions thought to represent the causes of a psychopathology and then measuring changes in the animals' behavior or physiology. The ethics of exposing animals to conditions that we would not expose humans to can be questioned, as can the generalizability of animal studies.

VI. Cross-cultural research

A. Cross-cultural research has expanded greatly in recent decades.

B. Some special challenges of cross-cultural research include difficulty in accessing populations, in applying theories appropriate in one culture to other cultures, in translating concepts and measures across cultures, in predicting the responses of people in different cultures to being studied, and in demands to define "healthy" and "unhealthy" cultures.

VII. Meta-analysis

A. Meta-analysis is a statistical technique for summarizing the results across several studies.

B. In a meta-analysis, the results of individual studies are standardized into a statistic called the effect size. Then the magnitude of the effect size and its relationship to characteristics of the study are examined.

C. Meta-analyses reduce bias that can occur when investigators draw conclusions across studies in a more subjective manner, but can include studies that have poor methods, and can exclude good studies that were not published because they did not find significant effects.

KEY TERMS AND GUIDED REVIEW

<u>Guided Review</u>

1. What are some of the challenges faced by researchers in abnormal psychology?

The Scientific Method

<u>Key Terms</u>

scientific method:

hypothesis:

null hypothesis:

variable:

dependent variable:

independent variable:

operationalization:

<u>Guided Review</u>

1. What is the difference between a primary hypothesis and a null hypothesis?

2. If the results of a study do not support the primary hypothesis, why does this not disprove the theory upon which the primary hypothesis is based?

3. What is the difference between an independent and dependent variable?

Case Studies

<u>Key Terms</u>

case study:

generalizability:

replication:

<u>Guided Review</u>

1. Suppose you wanted to test the hypothesis that a lack of aerobic exercise causes depression. How would you design a case study to test this hypothesis?

2. What are some advantages and disadvantages of case studies?

Correlational Studies

<u>Key Terms</u>

correlational study:

continuous variable:

group comparison study:

cross-sectional:

longitudinal:

correlation coefficient:

statistical significance:

third variable problem:

sample:

external validity:

<u>Guided Review</u>

1. What advantages and disadvantages do longitudinal studies have compared to cross-sectional studies?

2. What is the difference between a positive and negative correlation?

3. How do researchers decide if a correlation is meaningful?

4. Why does correlation not imply causation?

5. Why is it important to have a representative sample, and what is an effective method of achieving a representative sample?

6. In a correlational study, how can researchers protect against the third variable problem?

7. What are some advantages and disadvantages of correlational studies?

Epidemiological Studies

Key Terms

epidemiology:

prevalence:

incidence:

risk factors:

Guided Review

1. What is the difference between the prevalence of a disorder and the incidence of a disorder?

2. What are some advantages and disadvantages of epidemiological studies?

Experimental Studies

Key Terms

experimental studies:

human laboratory study:

analogue study:

internal validity:

control group:

experimental group:

random assignment:

demand characteristics:

therapy outcome study:

wait list control group:

placebo control group:

double-blind experiment:

efficacy:

effectiveness:

single-case experimental design:

ABAB design:

reversal design:

animal studies:

<u>Guided Review</u>

1. What is the difference between internal and external validity?

2. How can researchers increase the internal validity of an experiment?

3. How can researchers guard against demand characteristics?

4. What are some advantages and disadvantages of human laboratory studies?

5. Why would a researcher use a wait list control group instead of a regular control group?

6. What are some advantages and disadvantages of placebo control groups?

7. What are some advantages and disadvantages of therapy outcome studies?

8. What are some advantages and disadvantages of single-case experimental designs?

9. What are some advantages and disadvantages of animal studies?

Cross-Cultural Research

<u>Guided Review</u>

1. Give an example of why researchers should be cautious in applying theories developed in one culture to individuals from another culture.

2. What are some of the difficulties encountered by cross-cultural researchers?

3. What are some advantages of conducting cross-cultural research?

Meta-analysis

<u>Key Terms</u>

meta-analysis:

<u>Guided Review</u>

1. Explain how a meta-analysis is conducted, and describe how an effect size statistic provides information about multiple studies.

2. What are some advantages and disadvantages of meta-analysis?

CHAPTER TEST

A. <u>Multiple Choice</u>. Choose the **best answer** to each question below.

1. If a researcher is studying the effects of humor on depression, depression is the:

    A. hypothesis.
    B. independent variable.
    C. dependent variable.
    D. operationalization.

Use the following study to answer questions 2 and 3:
Professor Cole believes that depression is caused by experiences of loss (e.g., death of a loved one, or the breakup of a relationship). She administers questionnaires that ask people about their experiences of loss and current depressive symptoms. She finds that depression and loss are not associated with one another in her study.

2. In this study, the questionnaires used to measure loss and depressive symptoms are the:

A. independent and dependent variables.
B. operationalization.
C. primary hypothesis.
D. null hypothesis.

3. The results of the study above fail to support the
A. primary hypothesis.
B. null hypothesis.
C. operationalization.
D. variables.

4. Which of the following is not an advantage of case studies?

A. They capture the uniqueness of an individual.
B. They help generate new ideas and provide tentative support for those ideas.
C. They are sometimes the only way to study rare problems.
D. They are very likely to be replicated.

5. Researchers administer measures of memory and social skills to incoming college students during their orientation to a university. They predict that better social skills will be associated with better memory. This type of study is a

A. group comparison study.
B. longitudinal study.
C. human laboratory study.
D. correlational study.

6. Researchers studying the relationship between success in college and frequency of alcohol use find that questionnaires measuring these variables are correlated -.45, $p < .05$. This means that

A. as alcohol use increases, success in college tends to decrease, and this finding is likely not due to chance alone.
B. as alcohol use decreases, success in college tends to decrease, but this finding is likely due to chance alone.
C. as success in college increases, alcohol use also increases, and these findings are likely not due to chance alone.
D. there is no relationship between success in college and alcohol use because the correlation is not statistically significant.

7. Which of the following is not an advantage of correlational studies?

A. The fact that they can be cross-sectional or longitudinal.
B. Their ability to establish that one variable causes another.
C. Their external validity.
D. The fact that they involve fewer ethical concerns than most experimental studies.

8. State University issued a press release indicating that 2 percent of their students developed an eating disorder for the first time during the last academic year. This refers to the _____ of eating disorders at State University.

    A. incidence
    B. lifetime prevalence
    C. 12-month prevalence
    D. risk factors

9. Professor Adams wants to study the relationship between anger and aggression. She brings research participants into the laboratory and has one group of them watch an anger-inducing video, while the other group watches a neutral video about making cheesecake. She then gives participants the opportunity to punch an inflatable doll if they wish. Participants who watched the anger video punch the doll more than participants who watched the cheesecake video. A problem with the internal validity of this study is that

    A. the sample was not randomly drawn from the population.
    B. the level of generalizability to real-world conditions is questionable.
    C. there is no control group.
    D. random assignment was not used.

10. An advantage of both human laboratory and therapy outcome studies is that

    A. they do not involve statistical significance tests.
    B. they have good internal validity.
    C. they involve very few ethical issues.
    D. they do not involve random assignment to condition.

11. Filler measures and cover stories are used to

    A. increase external validity.
    B. prevent demand effects.
    C. increase demand effects.
    D. increase internal validity.

12. Which of the following statements is true?

    A. If the results of a study fail to support the null hypothesis, then the primary hypothesis has been proven.
    B. If two variables are correlated .99, $p < .05$, then we know that one variable causes the other.
    C. Results that are not statistically significant support the null hypothesis.
    D. Variables must be operationalized before being defined.

13. Which of the following cannot establish causal relationships?

A. Correlational studies
B. Animal studies
C. Human laboratory studies
D. Therapy outcome studies

14. Which of the following is used to increase external validity?

A. Statistical significance tests
B. Random assignment
C. Matching
D. Random sampling

15. To rule out third variables, a researcher should

A. use statistical significance tests.
B. conduct a longitudinal study.
C. use random assignment.
D. attempt to increase external validity.

16. A disadvantage of a single-case experimental design is

A. that it does not provide information about causation.
B. that it allows for intensive investigation of participants.
C. that the results may not generalize to the wider population.
D. the third-variable problem.

17. The use of which of the following is most controversial in therapy outcome studies?

A. Matching
B. Placebo control groups
C. Random sampling
D. Demand characteristics

18. Which of the following is not a basic right of research participants?

A. Participants must receive something tangible for their participation (e.g., money or lottery tickets).
B. Information collected during the study will be kept confidential.
C. Participants may choose to not participate in the study.
D. The purpose of the research should be explained to participants at the end of the study.

19. The file drawer effect refers to

A. the difficulty in comparing studies from different researchers.
B. researchers filing away studies that do not support the investigator's hypothesis.
C. the tendency of researchers to forget about older studies.

D. demand characteristics that often affect the performance of college student research participants.

20. Which of the following statements about Janice Egeland's study of the Amish is <u>true</u>?

    A. The Amish varied greatly in education and income status and were therefore difficult to study.
    B. The manifestations of depression and mania were different among the Amish as compared to mainstream society.
    C. The Amish were poor candidates for genetic studies of mood disorders, although much was still learned by studying them.
    D. The researchers violated ethical guidelines by studying the Amish because they did not wish to be studied by outsiders.

B. <u>True-False</u>. Select T (True) or F (False) below.

1. If intelligence and drug use are correlated -.70, $p > .05$, then we know that a statistically significant relationship exists between these variables.   T   F
2. The prevalence of a disorder refers to the number of individuals who develop a disorder during a specific time period.   T   F

3. Low internal validity is a problem with case studies, cross-sectional studies, and longitudinal studies.   T   F

4. Random assignment is important for establishing external validity, whereas random sampling is important for internal validity.   T   F

5. A treatment's efficacy refers to how well the treatment works in a highly controlled setting with a well-defined group of patients.   T   F

C. <u>Short Answer Questions</u>.

1. What are some ethical issues involved in conducting human laboratory, therapy outcome, and animal studies?

2. Describe some difficulties in conducting cross-cultural research.

3. Compare and contrast the benefits of conducting case studies, correlational research, and human laboratory research.

4. Why is it important to conduct statistical significance tests?

5. Describe some methods of controlling for demand characteristics in a study.

ANSWER KEY

Multiple Choice
1. C
2. B
3. A
4. D
5. D
6. A
7. B
8. A
9. C
10. B
11. B
12. C
13. A
14. D
15. C
16. C
17. D
18. A
19. B
20. B

True-False
1. F
2. F
3. T
4. F
5. F

Short Answer Questions
1. See pp. 84-89.
2. See pp. 90-91.
3. See pp. 74-85.
4. See p. 78-79.
5. See p. 83-84.

Additional Readings on Chapter 3 Topics
    Faust, D., & Meehl, P. E. (1992). Using scientific methods to resolve questions in the history and philosophy of science: Some illustrations. Behavior Therapy, 23, 195-211.
    Wampold, B. E., Davis, B., & Good, R. H. (1990). Hypothesis validity of clinical research. Journal of Consulting and Clinical Psychology, 58, 360-367.
    Wilkinson, L. (1999). Statistical methods in psychology journals: Guidelines and explanations. American Psychologist, 54, 594-604.

Chapter 4: Assessing and Diagnosing Abnormality

LEARNING OBJECTIVES

After reading and studying this chapter, you should be able to:

1. Discuss the types of information that should be obtained during an assessment, and why each is important in ensuring that clinicians gather all the information that is needed for an accurate assessment.

2. Describe and give examples of each of the various tools used by clinicians to gather information during an assessment. Discuss the advantages and disadvantages of each assessment tool.

3. Define and distinguish among the various psychometric properties (i.e., reliability and validity) that set the standard by which various assessment tools are evaluated.

4. Discuss the problems in assessment, and how they might be overcome or diminished.

5. Discuss the modern method for diagnosing mental disorders, the DSM-IV, and discuss its five axes.

6. Discuss the changes in the DSM from its earliest version to its most recent version, and the factors that have influenced the changes.

7. Discuss the dangers inherent in diagnosing a person with a mental disorder.

ESSENTIAL IDEAS

I. Gathering information

    A. Information concerning clients' symptoms and history is obtained in an assessment. This information includes the details of their current symptoms, ability to function, coping strategies, recent events, history of psychological problems, and family history of psychological problems.

    B. Clients' physiological and neurophysiological functioning is assessed as well. Clients may be asked to undergo a physical examination to detect medical conditions, questioned about their drug use, and tested for their cognitive functioning and intellectual abilities.

    C. Clients' sociocultural background—including their social resources and cultural heritage—are important to ascertain in an assessment.

II. Assessment tools

A. Paper-and-pencil neuropsychological tests can help to identify specific cognitive deficits that may be tied to brain damage.

B. CT, PET, and MRI technologies are currently being used to investigate the structural and functional differences between the brains of people with psychological disorders and those of people without disorders. We cannot yet use these technologies to diagnose specific psychological disorders in individual patients.

C. Intelligence tests can indicate a client's general level of intellectual functioning in verbal and analytic tasks.

D. Structured interviews provide a standardized way to assess, in an interview format, people's symptoms.

E. Symptom questionnaires allow for mass screening of large numbers of people to determine self-reported symptoms.

F. Personality inventories assess stable personality characteristics.

G. Projective tests are used to uncover unconscious conflicts and concerns but are open to interpretive biases.

H. Behavioral observation and self-monitoring can help detect behavioral deficits and the environmental triggers for symptoms.

III. Problems in assessment

A. It is often difficult to obtain accurate information on children's problems because children are unable to report their thoughts and feelings. Parents and teachers may provide information about children, but they can be biased in their own assessments of children's symptoms and needs.

B. When the clinician and client are from different cultures, language difficulties and cultural expectations can make assessment difficult. Interpreters can help in the assessment process but must be well-trained in psychological assessment.

IV. Diagnosis

A. The <u>Diagnostic and Statistical Manual of Mental Disorders</u> (DSM) provides criteria for diagnosing all psychological disorders currently recognized in the United States.

B. The first two editions of the DSM provided vague descriptions of disorders based on psychoanalytic theory; thus, the reliability of diagnoses made according to these manuals was low. More recent editions of the DSM contain more specific, observable criteria that are not as strongly based on theory for the diagnosis of disorders.

C. Five axes, or dimensions, of information are specified in determining a DSM diagnosis:

On Axis I, clinicians list all significant clinical syndromes.

On Axis II, clinicians indicate if the client is suffering from a personality disorder or mental retardation.

On Axis III, clinicians list the client's general medical condition.

On Axis IV, clinicians list psychosocial and environmental problems the client is facing.

On Axis V, clinicians indicate the client's global level of functioning.

D. Many critics of the DSM argue that it reflects Western, male perspectives on abnormality and pathologizes the behavior of women and other cultures. The DSM-IV includes descriptions of culture-bound syndromes—groups of symptoms that appear to occur only in specific cultures.

E. Diagnoses can be misapplied for political or social reasons. The negative social implications of having a psychiatric diagnosis can be great, but having a standard diagnostic system helps in treatment and research.

KEY TERMS AND GUIDED REVIEW

<u>Key Terms</u>

assessment:

diagnosis:

Gathering Information

<u>Key Terms</u>

differential diagnosis:

acculturation:

<u>Guided Review</u>

1. In addition to finding out which symptoms a client has, what additional information should be gathered in an assessment?

2. What is the appropriate role of biological tests in psychological assessment?

3. Why is making a differential diagnosis important?

4. Why is it important to determine a client's level of acculturation?

Assessment Tools

<u>Key Terms</u>

unstructured interview:

structured interview:

resistance:

validity:

face validity:

content validity:

concurrent validity:

predictive validity:

construct validity:

reliability:

test-retest reliability:

alternate form reliability:

internal reliability:

interrater reliability:

neuropsychological tests:

computerized tomography (CT):

positron-emission tomography (PET):

magnetic resonance imaging (MRI):

intelligence tests:

symptom questionnaire:

personality inventories:

projective test:

behavioral observation:

self-monitoring:

Guided Review

1. What are the advantages and disadvantages of unstructured interviews, compared to structured interviews?

2. What is the difference between validity and reliability?

3. What are some reasons for using neuropsychological tests in assessment?

4. How are CT, PET, and MRI different from one another?

5. What are some reasons for using intelligence tests in an assessment?

6. What are some of the criticisms of intelligence tests?

7. Why are symptom questionnaires useful?

8. What are some advantages and disadvantages of the MMPI?

9. Give some examples of projective tests and what they are thought to measure. What are some limitations of projective tests?

10. What are some advantages and disadvantages of using behavioral observations in an assessment?

Problems in Assessment

Guided Review

1. When assessing a child, what are some reasons for obtaining information from people besides the child him/herself?

2. What problems can result from using parents to assess a child's functioning?

3. What problems can result from using teachers to assess a child's functioning?

4. What are some difficulties that can arise when assessing a client from another culture?

Diagnosis

Key Terms

syndrome:

classification system:

Diagnostic and Statistical Manual of Mental Disorders (DSM):

Guided Review

1. How do psychological syndromes differ from medical syndromes?

2. What are some of the ways in which the DSM changed from its first edition in 1952 through publication of its fourth edition in 1994?

3. What are some reasons why the DSM does not have perfect reliability?

4. Summarize the information that should appear on Axes I through V of the DSM.

5. What are some criticisms of the DSM-IV?

6. What are some of the advantages and disadvantages of using diagnostic labels?

7. What did Rosenhan's (1973) study illustrate about the dangers of diagnostic labels?

CHAPTER TEST

A. Multiple Choice. Choose the **best answer** to each question below.

1. Clinicians do not use biological tests

    A. to determine if a person is suffering from a medical condition that causes psychological symptoms.
    B. to determine if a patient has a brain injury or tumor.
    C. to identify gross structural or functional abnormalities in an individual patient.
    D. to make a differential diagnosis between two mental disorders in an individual patient.

2. All of the following are particularly important for making a differential diagnosis except

    A. recent events in the client's life.
    B. the client's past history of psychological problems.
    C. the client's self-concept and concept of his or her symptoms.

D. the client's family history of psychological problems.

3. The extent to which a test yields the same results as other measures of the same behavior, thoughts, or feelings is referred to as

    A. test-retest reliability.
    B. predictive validity.
    C. concurrent validity.
    D. construct validity.

4. Similarity in people's answers to different parts of the same test is referred to as

    A. test-retest reliability.
    B. internal reliability.
    C. alternate form reliability.
    D. face validity.

5. Which of the following involves passing narrow X-ray beams through a person's head, determining the amount of radiation absorbed by each beam, and then constructing a computerized 3-D image of the person's brain?

    A. CT
    B. MRI
    C. PET
    D. EEG

6. An IQ score of 100 means that

    A. the client's intellectual abilities are in the mentally retarded range.
    B. the client's intellectual abilities are in the gifted range.
    C. the client's intellectual abilities are in the average range.
    D. the IQ test is not appropriate for the client being tested.

7. Which of the following statements about the BDI is <u>true</u>?

    A. It can be used to diagnose depression.
    B. It discriminates clearly between the symptoms of depression and the symptoms of other disorders (e.g., anxiety disorders).
    C. It is useful in learning about an individual's unconscious motives.
    D. It has cutoff scores that indicate moderate and severe levels of depression.

8. The most widely used test of personality is the

    A. Bender-Gestalt Test
    B. Minnesota Multiphasic Personality Inventory
    C. Rorschach Inkblot Test

D. Draw-a-Person Test

9. The reliability and validity of _____ has not proven to be strong in research.

    A. neuropsychological tests
    B. intelligence tests
    C. personality inventories
    D. projective tests

10. Which of the following statements about assessing children is <u>false</u>?

    A. Children are typically able to differentiate among different types of emotions that they experience.
    B. Children with behavior problems often do not believe that they have problems.
    C. Parents' reports of child behavior may be affected by their own psychopathology.
    D. Teachers' assessments of children are often discrepant with the assessments given by parents and clinicians.

11. Which of the following statements about cultural biases in assessment is <u>false</u>?

    A. African Americans tend to be overdiagnosed with schizophrenia even when their symptoms actually fit the diagnosis of bipolar disorder.
    B. When the clinician and client do not speak the same language, the clinician is highly likely to overdiagnose symptomatology rather than underdiagnose it.
    C. European Americans are more likely than members of other cultures to report feeling anxious or sad, whereas members of some other cultures tend to report symptoms as physical complaints.
    D. Members of non-European cultures may tend to be overdiagnosed with psychotic symptoms when they are really reporting on the beliefs of their culture.

12. The DSM is considered a

    A. symptom questionnaire.
    B. self-monitoring system.
    C. syndrome.
    D. classification system.

13. From the DSM in 1952 to the DSM-IV in 1994, the trend in diagnostic criteria has been

    A. from vague, atheoretical classifications of disorders to theory-based criteria for each disorder.
    B. from not providing information about how long a person must display certain symptoms in order to qualify for a diagnosis to providing this information.
    C. from including prevalence information to concluding that cross-cultural differences make such information unsound.
    D. from requiring that symptoms either cause distress or interfere with functioning to

requiring that unconscious conflicts play a role in the development of disorders.

14. Beginning with its third edition, the DSM was revamped due to

    A. problems with the validity of diagnostic criteria.
    B. insufficient theory regarding the causes of disorders in earlier editions.
    C. problems with the reliability of diagnostic criteria.
    D. the requirement (in earlier editions) that one's symptoms interfere with functioning.

15. Mental retardation should be coded on

    A. Axis I.
    B. Axis II.
    C. Axis III.
    D. Axis IV.

16. Problems such as housing or economic difficulties should be recorded on

    A. Axis IV.
    B. Axis II.
    C. Axis V.
    D. Axis III.

17. A client whose Global Assessment of Functioning (GAF) is 90 would be regarded as having

    A. some danger of hurting self or others or gross impairment in communication.
    B. moderate symptoms and difficulty in functioning.
    C. serious symptoms and difficulty in functioning.
    D. absent or minimal symptoms; good functioning in all areas.

18. Some researchers argue that diagnosis should be based on a _____ approach, rather than the current use of discrete categories of disorders.

    A. dimensional
    B. subjective
    C. numerical
    D. case-by-case

19. Which individual has argued that mental disorders do not really exist?

    A. David Rosenhan
    B. Thomas Szasz
    C..Hippocrates
    D. Hermann Rorschach

20. The research conducted by Harris and colleagues (1992) illustrated

A. sex bias in diagnosis.
B. cultural bias in diagnosis.
C. negative implications of diagnostic labels.
D. the low reliability of diagnostic labels.

B. <u>True-False</u>. Select T (True) or F (False) below.

1. Construct validity is the extent to which a test assesses all the important aspects of a phenomenon that it purports to measure.   T   F

2. Alternate form reliability is an index of how consistent the results of a test are over time.   T   F

3. The Bender-Gestalt Test is an example of a projective test.   T   F

4. Magnetic Resonance Imaging (MRI) does not require exposing a patient to any form of radiation, but Positron Emission Tomograpy (PET) does.   T   F

5. The Beck Depression Inventory (BDI) cannot establish a diagnosis of depression.   T   F

C. <u>Short Answer Questions</u>.

1. Identify five areas that are important to assess during a clinical interview. For each area, briefly explain why it is important to assess and give an example of how you might assess it.

2. Give a brief description of CT scans, PET, and MRI.

3. Discuss how cultural biases can affect the assessment process. Give some examples from the chapter.

4. What are some of the shortcomings of the DSM-IV-TR? How does the DSM-IV-TR represent an improvement over earlier versions of the DSM?

5. What are the advantages and disadvantages of using diagnostic labels?

ANSWER KEY

<u>Multiple Choice</u>
1. D
2. C
3. C
4. B
5. A
6. C
7. D
8. B
9. D
10. A
11. B
12. D
13. B
14. C
15. B
16. A
17. D
18. A
19. B
20. C

<u>True-False</u>
1. F
2. F
3. F
4. T
5. T

<u>Short Answer Questions</u>
1. See p. 104.
2. See pp. 107–108.
3. See pp. 117–118.
4. See pp. 119–125.
5. See pp. 125–127.

Additional Readings on Chapter 4 Topics

Beutler, L. E., & Malik, M. L. (2002). <u>Rethinking the DSM: A psychological perspective</u>. Washington, DC: American Psychological Association.

Cipolotti, L., & Warrington, E. K. (1995). Neuropsychological assessment. <u>Journal of Neurology, Neurosurgery, and Psychiatry, 58,</u> 655-664.

Garb, H. N. (1997). Race bias, social class bias, and gender bias in clinical judgment. <u>Clinical Psychology: Science and Practice, 4,</u> 99-120.

Chapter 5: Treatments for Abnormality

LEARNING OBJECTIVES

After reading and studying this chapter, you should be able to:

1. Give examples of antipsychotic, antidepressant, mood stabilizing, and antianxiety drugs and know their appropriate uses and limitations.

2. Distinguish among MAO inhibitors, tricyclic antidepressants, and SSRIs.

3. Identify the appropriate and inappropriate uses of ECT, psychosurgery, and repetitive transcranial magnetic stimulation (rTMS).

4. Give examples of herbal remedies for the treatment of psychological problems and discuss what is known about their effectiveness.

5. Describe the components of psychodynamic therapy and how it is thought to work.

6. Describe humanistic therapy and how it is conducted.

7. Describe techniques used in behavior therapy.

8. Describe the elements of cognitive therapy and how it is similar to behavior therapy.

9. Discuss IPT and how it is both similar to and different from psychodynamic therapy.

10. Discuss alternatives to individual therapy (e.g., family and group therapy).

11. Describe how mental health treatment may be carried out in the community.

12. Discuss how cultural issues may affect treatment and the extent to which research suggests that these issues should affect therapist-client matching.

13. Summarize the common components of successful therapies.

14. Discuss the special issues that can arise when treating children.

ESSENTIAL IDEAS

I. Biological treatments

    A. Antipsychotic drugs, such as phenothiazines and butyrophenone, help reduce the symptoms of psychosis.

B. Antidepressant drugs, including the monoamine oxidase inhibitors, the tricyclic antidepressants, and the selective serotonin reuptake inhibitors help reduce the symptoms of depression.

C. Lithium is used to treat the symptoms of mania.

D. Anticonvulsant drugs and calcium channel blockers also help to treat mania.

E. Antianxiety drugs include the barbiturates and the benzodiazepines.

F. Herbal medicines are popular but the efficacy and safety of some of these drugs has not been definitively shown.

G. Electroconvulsive therapy (ECT) is useful in treating severe depression.

H. Psychosurgery is used on rare occasions to help people with severe psychopathology that is not affected by drugs or other treatments.

I. Repetitive transcranial magnetic stimulation (rTMS) is a new technique that involves exposing the brain to magnets. It may be helpful in the treatment of depression.

II. Psychological therapies

A. Psychodynamic therapies focus on uncovering unconscious motives and concerns behind psychopathology through free association and analysis of transferences and dreams.

B. Humanistic, or client-centered, therapy attempts to help clients find their own answers to problems by supporting them and reflecting back these concerns, so they can self-reflect and self-actualize.

C. Behavior therapies focus on altering the reinforcements and punishments people receive for maladaptive behavior. Behavior therapists also help clients learn new behavioral skills.

D. Cognitive therapy focuses on changing the maladaptive cognitions behind distressing feelings and behaviors.

III. Interpersonal and social approaches

A. Interpersonal therapy is a short-term therapy that focuses on clients' current relationships and concerns but explores the roots of their problems in past relationships.

B. Family systems therapists focus on changing maladaptive patterns of behavior within family systems to reduce psychopathology in individual members.

C. In group therapy, people who share a problem come together to support each other, learn from each other, and practice new skills. Self-help groups are a form of group therapy that does not involve a mental health professional.

D. The community mental health movement was aimed at deinstitutionalizing people with mental disorders and treating them through community mental health centers, halfway houses, and day treatment centers. The resources for these community treatment centers have never been adequate, however, and many people do not have access to mental health care.

E. Primary prevention programs aim to stop the development of disorders before they start.

F. Secondary prevention programs provide treatment to people in the early stages of their disorders in the hope of reducing the development of the disorders.

G. The values inherent in most psychotherapies that can clash with the values of certain cultures include the focus on the individual, the expression of emotions and disclosure of personal concerns, and the expectation that clients take initiative.

H. People from minority groups may be more likely to remain in treatment if matched with a therapist from their own cultural group, but there are large individual differences in these preferences.

I. There are a number of culturally specific therapies designed by cultural groups to address psychopathology within the traditions of those cultures.

IV. Evaluating treatments

A. Some reviews of studies of the effectiveness of psychosocial treatments find they are all equally effective, but others suggest that certain treatments are more effective than others in treating specific disorders.

B. Methodological and ethical problems make doing good research on the effectiveness of therapy difficult.

C. Most successful therapies establish a positive relationship between a therapist and client, provide an explanation or interpretation to the client, and encourage the client to confront painful emotions.

V. Special issues in treating children

A. Treatments for children must take into account their cognitive skills and developmental levels and must adapt to their ability to comprehend and participate in therapy.

B. There are reasons to be concerned about the possible toxic effects of prescription drugs on children.

C. Often, a child's family must be brought into therapy, but the child or the family may object.

D. Most children who enter therapy do not seek it out themselves but are taken by others, raising issues about children's willingness to participate in therapy.

KEY TERMS AND GUIDED REVIEW

<u>Key Terms</u>

psychotherapy:

Biological Treatments

<u>Key Terms</u>

chlorpromazine:

phenothiazines:

neuroleptic:

butyrophenone:

antipsychotic drugs:

antidepressants:

monoamine oxidase inhibitors (MAOIs):

tricyclic antidepressants:

selective serotonin reuptake inhibitor (SSRI):

lithium:

anticonvulsants:

calcium channel blockers:

antianxiety drugs:

barbiturates:

benzodiazepines:

electroconvulsive therapy (ECT):

prefrontal lobotomy:

psychosurgery:

repetitive transcranial magnetic stimulation (rTMS)

Guided Review

1. Discuss how the first antipsychotic drugs were discovered.

2. Describe some of the differences between MAOIs, tricyclic antidepressants, and SSRIs.

3. What are some reasons why SSRIs have become so popular?

4. List the side effects of MAOIs, tricyclic antidepressants, SSRIs, barbiturates, and benzodiazepines.

5. Discuss how lithium was discovered to be an effective treatment for mania.

6. Describe some advantages and disadvantages of using St. John's Wort for the treatment of depression.

7. Discuss what is known about the effectiveness of herbal medicines for the treatment of anxiety.

8. Describe how ECT is performed in the modern age.

9. Describe some potential advantages of using rTMS for the treatment of depression.

10. Discuss the impact of the introduction of drug therapies for psychological problems on society.

Psychological Therapies

Key Terms

psychodynamic therapies:

free association:

resistance:

transference:

working through:

catharsis:

therapeutic alliance:

psychoanalysis:

humanistic therapy:

person-centered therapy:

client-centered therapy:

unconditional positive regard:

reflection:

behavior therapies:

behavioral assessment:

role play:

systematic desensitization therapy:

modeling:

in vivo exposure:

flooding:

implosive therapy:

token economy:

response shaping:

social skills training:

cognitive therapies:

behavioral assignments:

<u>Guided Review</u>

1. What are some of the main components of psychodynamic therapy, and how is it thought to work?

2. What is the difference between psychoanalysis and psychodynamic therapy?

3. What are some limitations of psychodynamic therapy?

4. What are the main components of client-centered therapy, and how is it thought to work?

5. What are some differences between client-centered therapy and psychodynamic therapy?

5. Describe how a behavior therapist might go about reducing unwanted behaviors in a client.

6. Describe how a behavior therapist might go about increasing positive behaviors in a client.

8. What are some goals of cognitive therapy?

9. Describe some techniques used by cognitive therapists.

10. In what ways are psychodynamic, humanistic, client-centered, behavioral, and cognitive therapies similar to and different from one another?

Interpersonal and social approaches

<u>Key Terms</u>

interpersonal therapy (IPT):

family systems therapy:

group therapy:

self-help groups:

community mental-health centers:

halfway houses:

day treatment centers:

primary prevention:

secondary prevention:

<u>Guided Review</u>

1. What are some similarities and differences between IPT and traditional psychodynamic therapy?

2. What are some similarities and differences between Minuchin's Structural Family Therapy and Satir's Conjoint Family Therapy?

3. What are the primary strategies of family therapy?

4. What advantages might group therapy have over individual therapy?

5. List and describe some alternatives to institutionalization for mental health patients.

6. What is the difference between primary and secondary prevention?

7. What are some ways in which non-Western cultural norms can clash with assumptions of psychotherapy?

8. What has recent research revealed about the importance of matching therapists and clients on variables such as gender and ethnicity?

9. Give some examples of culturally specific therapies.

Evaluating Treatments

<u>Guided Review</u>

1. What appear to be some common components of successful therapies?

Special Issues in Treating Children

<u>Guided Review</u>

1. Give an example of how a therapy developed for adults may be applied differently with children.

2. What are some safety issues that arise when treating a child's psychopathology with drugs?

3. What are some difficulties that arise when treating children using psychotherapy?

CHAPTER TEST

A. Multiple Choice. Choose the **best answer** to each question below.

1. Chlorpromazine belongs to the group of drugs known as

> A. tricyclic antidepressants.
> B. monoamine oxidase inhibitors.
> C. phenothiazines.
> D. butyrophenones.

2. Tardive dyskinesia is a side effect that may be caused by

> A. tricyclic antidepressants.
> B. phenothiazines.
> C. lithium.
> D. benzodiazepines.

3. Inhibiting monoamine oxidase

> A. leads to lower levels of dopamine in the synapse.
> B. inhibits the reuptake of serotonin.
> C. leads to higher levels of norepinephrine in the synapse.
> D. increases levels of substance P.

4. One important reason that selective serotonin reuptake inhibitors (SSRIs) became very popular soon after their development was

> A. they were shown to be more effective than tricyclic antidepressants.
> B. they were shown to be more effective than MAO inhibitors.
> C. they were found to be specific to depression and not other problems.
> D. their side effects were more easily tolerated by many people.

5. _____ may be prescribed to treat mania.

> A. Calcium channel blockers
> B. Benzodiazepines
> C. Barbiturates
> D. MAO inhibitors

6. Which of the following appears to be an effective treatment for mild to moderate depression?

    A. Hypericum perforatum
    B. Rauwolfia serpentina
    C. Valeriana officinalis
    D. Gingko biloba

7. Research has found repetitive transcranial magnetic stimulation to reduce _____ and _____.

    A. seizures; impulsiveness
    B. anxiety; depression
    C. mania; seizures
    D. depression; auditory hallucinations

8. Analyzing a client's transference toward the therapist would most likely occur in

    A. behavior therapy.
    B. psychodynamic therapy.
    C. cognitive therapy.
    D. client-centered therapy.

9. Exposing clients to feared stimuli or situations to an excessive degree while preventing them from avoiding the stimuli or situation is known as

    A. modeling.
    B. systematic desensitization.
    C. response shaping.
    D. flooding.

10. Reflection is a therapeutic method used in _____ therapy.

    A. behavioral
    B. psychodynamic
    C. client-centered
    D. cognitive

11. A key technique used by humanistic therapists is

    A. allowing a client to freely convey his or her thoughts and feelings in an unstructured manner, collecting bits of information from these thoughts, and eventually voicing an interpretation about the client's problems.
    B. changing the client's tendency to automatically assume that his or her negative thoughts are true by identifying and challenging them.
    C. communicating to the client that the therapist is a real person like the client, and can empathize with the client's concerns in a nondirective way.

D. focusing on the client's relationships as the source of his or her distress while voicing interpretations and directing the client toward changing these relationships.

12. A therapy that focuses on pointing out dysfunctional communication patterns in families and teaching family members to communicate better is known as

    A. interpersonal therapy (IPT).
    B. Satir's conjoint family therapy.
    C. Yalom's group therapy.
    D. Minuchin's structural family therapy.

13. A place where people with long-standing mental health problems may live in a structured, supportive environment is known as a

    A. community mental health center.
    B. halfway house.
    C. day treatment program.
    D. homebuilders program.

14. Approximately _____ percent of people with a severe mental illness do not receive any mental health care.

    A. 10
    B. 25
    C. 50
    D. 85

15. Research on social factors has not shown that

    A. matching therapist and client on ethnicity or race leads to better outcomes for the client.
    B. people from Latino, Asian, and Native American cultures are more comfortable with structured and action-oriented therapies than with less structured therapies.
    C. people from ethnic minority groups in the U.S. are more likely to drop out of psychotherapy.
    D. men and women report that they prefer a therapist of the same gender.

16. All of the following have been found to be common components of successful therapies except:

    A. a positive relationship with the therapist.
    B. an explanation or interpretation of why the client is suffering.
    C. short-term, structured therapy sessions.
    D. confrontation of negative emotions.

17. In 1952, Hans Eysenck concluded that

A. psychotherapy was effective for a wide variety of problems.
B. behavior therapies were superior to psychodynamic therapies for most disorders.
C. all therapies were about equally effective.
D. psychotherapy did not work.

18. The Dodo bird verdict states that

A. all psychotherapies have not been shown to be effective.
B. drug therapies are equivalent to psychotherapies in their effectiveness.
C. no psychotherapy has been convincingly shown to be more effective than another.
D. all psychotherapies have been shown to be effective.

19. Which of the following is not a problem in treating children?

A. Children cannot participate meaningfully in talking therapies, such as cognitive therapy.
B. Studies of the long-term impact of drugs on child development have not been done.
C. Children often do not seek therapy themselves.
D. There is more variability in the proper dosage of a drug among children than there is among adults.

20. An eclectic therapist

A. practices only those techniques that have been shown to be effective.
B. uses techniques of different therapies depending on the specific issues needing to be addressed.
C. believes that drug therapies should be the treatment of choice for most disorders.
D. receives extensive training in one therapy from an expert and practices only that form of therapy.

B. True-False. Select T (True) or F (False) below.

1. Most antipsychotic drugs are thought to work by increasing norepinephrine levels or influencing receptors for norepinephrine in the brain.   T   F

2. Self-help groups often utilize approaches from client-centered therapy.   T   F

3. Anticonvulsants and calcium channel blockers are effective treatments for depression.
          T   F

4. The notion of unconditional positive regard was introduced by Freud.   T   F

5. Both interpersonal therapy and cognitive therapy are designed to be short-term treatments.

    T   F

C. Short Answer Questions.

1. How does the role of the therapist differ in psychodynamic therapy as compared to cognitive therapy?

2. Why are SSRIs preferred over MAOIs and tricyclic antidepressants?

3. What are some common components of successful therapies?

4. What are some reasons that therapies developed in Western cultures may be hard to practice with individuals from different cultures?

5. Describe some special considerations that should be made when treating children.

ANSWER KEY

<u>Multiple Choice</u>
1. D
2. B
3. C
4. D
5. A
6. A
7. D
8. B
9. D
10. C
11. C
12. B
13. B
14. C
15. A
16. C
17. D
18. C
19. A
20. B

<u>True-False</u>
1. F
2. T
3. F
4. F
5. T

<u>Short Answer Questions</u>
1. See pp. 145–147, 151–154.
2. See pp. 138–139.
3. See pp. 163–164.
4. See pp. 159–161.
5. See pp. 164–167.

Additional Reading on Chapter 5 Topics

Chambless, D. L., & Ollendick, T. H. (2000). Empirically supported psychological interventions: Controversies and evidence. Annual Review of Psychology, 52, 685-716.

Elkin, I. A. (1999). A major dilemma in psychotherapy outcome research: Disentangling therapists from therapies. Clinical Psychology: Science and Practice, 6, 10-32.

Nathan, P. E., & Gorman, J. M. (2002). A guide to treatments that work: Second edition. New York: Oxford University Press.

Chapter 6: Stress Disorders and Health Psychology

LEARNING OBJECTIVES
After reading and studying this chapter, you should be able to:

1. Discuss the characteristics of events that people perceive as stressful.

2. Describe the fight-or-flight response and the phases of the general adaptation syndrome.

3. Define health psychology and discuss the three predominant models for how psychological factors affect physical disease.

4. Discuss the relationship between psychological factors and coronary heart disease, as well as hypertension.

5. Discuss how psychological factors can influence immune functioning and the evidence that psychological factors influence the development and course of physical illness.

6. Discuss the negative physiological and psychological effects of sleep deprivation.

7. Distinguish among the various sleep disorders, including dyssomnias, and parasomnias.

8. Discuss some of the treatments available for sleep disorders.

9. Explain how dispositional pessimism may contribute to physical illness, and describe the specific evidence that supports this view.

10. Distinguish between Type A and Type B personalities, and discuss the evidence that Type A personality is associated with early mortality and coronary heart disease.

11. Identify the specific aspects of Type A personality that are most detrimental to health.

12 Discuss the role of social support in health and describe the relations among marriage, gender, and physical health.

13. Describe the elements of guided mastery techniques, biofeedback, and support groups and discuss their effectiveness in improving physical health.

14. Summarize the symptoms of PTSD, acute stress disorder, and adjustment disorder.

15. Discuss the types of events that can contribute to PTSD.

16. Discuss the sociocultural, psychological, and biological factors associated with increased risk of PTSD.

17. Discuss treatments for PTSD, including systematic desensitization therapy, stress management techniques, eye movement desensitization and reprocessing, and biological approaches.

18. Discuss cross-cultural differences in the presentation and treatment of PTSD.

ESSENTIAL IDEAS

I. Physiological responses to stress

    A. The body has a natural response to stress that prepares it for fight or flight. In the short term, this response is highly adaptive, but if it is chronically aroused, it can cause physical damage.

    B. There is substantial evidence that stress, particularly uncontrollable stress, increases risks for coronary heart disease and hypertension, probably through chronic hyperarousal of the body's fight-or-flight response.

    C. There is mounting evidence from animal and human studies that stress impairs the functioning of the immune system, possibly leading to higher rates of infectious diseases.

II. Sleep and health

    A. The sleep disorders are divided into sleep disorders related to another mental disorder, sleep disorders due to a general medical condition, substance-induced sleep disorders, and primary sleep disorders.

    B. The primary sleep disorders are further divided into dyssomnias and parasomnias.

    C. The most common dyssomnia is insomnia. Hypersomnia, narcolepsy, and breathing-related sleep disorders, such as sleep apnea, are also dyssomnias.

    D. Sleep disorders, particularly insomnia, can be treated with a variety of drugs or through behavioral and cognitive-behavioral therapies that change sleep-related behavior and thinking patterns.

III. Personality and health

    A. People who are chronically pessimistic may show poorer physical health because they appraise more events as uncontrollable or because they engage in poorer health-related behaviors.

    B. People with the Type A behavior pattern are highly competitive, time urgent, and hostile. The Type A behavior pattern significantly increases the risk for coronary heart disease. The most potent component of this pattern is hostility, which alone significantly predicts heart disease.

C. People who receive high-quality social support have more positive physical health outcomes in stressful situations than those who have little social support or much social friction.

IV. Interventions to improve health

A. Guided mastery techniques help people learn positive health-related behaviors by teaching them the most effective ways of engaging in these behaviors and by giving them opportunities to practice the behaviors in increasingly challenging situations.

B. Biofeedback is used to help people learn to control their own negative physiological responses.

C. Support groups are one source of social support for some people. Some research suggests that they can improve both psychological and physical well-being.

V. Posttraumatic stress disorder and acute stress disorder

A. People with posttraumatic stress disorder repeatedly reexperience the traumatic event, avoid situations that might arouse memories of their trauma, and are hypervigilant and chronically aroused.

B. PTSD may be most likely to occur following traumas that shatter individuals' assumptions that they are invulnerable, that the world is a just place, and that bad things do not happen to good people.

C. People who experience severe and long-lasting traumas, who have lower levels of social support, who experience socially stigmatizing traumas, who were already depressed or anxious before the trauma, or who have maladaptive coping styles may be at increased risk for PTSD.

D. People who are unable to somehow make sense of a trauma appear more likely to have chronic PTSD symptoms.

E. PTSD sufferers show greater physiological reactivity to stressors, greater activity in areas of the brain involved in emotion and memory, but lower resting cortisol levels.

F. Effective psychotherapy for PTSD involves exposing the person to memories of the trauma and extinguishing his or her anxiety over these memories through systematic desensitization and flooding.

G. Some people cannot tolerate such exposure, however, and may do better with supportive therapy focused on solving current interpersonal difficulties and life problems.

H. Benzodiazepines and antidepressant drugs can quell some of the symptoms of PTSD.

I. Clinicians must be sensitive both to the extraordinary circumstances that may have led to PTSD and to the cultural norms of the person or group being treated.

KEY TERMS AND GUIDED REVIEW

Key Terms

stress:

Guided Review

1. Describe the direct effects, interactive, and indirect effects models.

Physiological Responses to Stress

Key Terms

fight-or-flight response:

cortisol:

general adaptation syndrome:

health psychology

coronary heart disease (CHD):

hypertension:

immune system:

lymphocytes:

Guided Review

1. What is the evidence that uncontrollable events are more stressful than controllable events?

2. Why do unpredictable events appear to be more stressful than predictable events?

3. Describe the fight-or-flight response.

4. Describe the phases of the general adaptation syndrome described by Selye.

5. How, according to Taylor and colleagues, do men and women differ in their responses to stressful events, and why do they differ?

6. Describe the models that explain how psychological factors impact physical disease and provide examples of each model.

7. Describe some contributors to coronary heart disease (CHD).

8. What is the evidence that stress is related to hypertension, and why are African Americans particularly prone to developing hypertension?

9. Give some research-based examples of how stress is related to immune functioning.

Sleep and Health

<u>Key Terms</u>

dyssomnias:

parasomnias:

insomnia:

stimulus control therapy:

sleep restriction therapy:

hypersomnia:

narcolepsy:

cataplexy:

sleep apnea:

<u>Guided Review</u>

1. Describe several of the negative health and safety effects of sleep deprivation.

2. What are some psychological effects of sleep deprivation?

3. In addition to simply getting more sleep, what are some ways that people can reduce sleepiness and sleep deprivation?

4. What are some of the medical conditions that can disturb sleep?

5. What must be present for someone to be diagnosed with insomnia?

6. Describe two ways that you could treat a patient with insomnia.

7. Describe the symptoms of hypersomnia.

8. What are the symptoms of narcolepsy and sleep apnea?

Personality and Health

<u>Key Terms</u>

Type A behavior pattern:

<u>Guided Review</u>

1. What is the evidence that pessimism is related to health?

2. What are some mechanisms through which pessimism is related to health?

3. Describe the Type A behavior pattern.

4. What is the evidence that the Type A behavior pattern is related to coronary heart disease (CHD)?

5. Which aspect(s) of Type A behavior appear to be most strongly related to negative health outcomes?

6. What are some mechanisms through which Type A behavior(s) may lead to CHD?

7. Describe how social support can be beneficial to health under some circumstances, but not others.

8. How are social support, gender, and health related to one another?

Interventions to Improve Health

<u>Key Terms</u>

guided mastery techniques:

biofeedback:

<u>Guided Review</u>

1. Give an example of a guided mastery technique. What is the evidence that these techniques are effective?

2. Describe biofeedback and some of its uses.

3. What are some limitations of biofeedback?

7. Describe some techniques that appear to be helpful for reducing Type A behavior.

8. What is the evidence that support groups are beneficial for physical health?

Posttraumatic Stress Disorder and Acute Stress Disorder

Key Terms

posttraumatic stress disorder (PTSD):

acute stress disorder:

dissociative symptoms:

adjustment disorder:

systematic desensitization therapy:

thought-stopping techniques:

stress-management interventions:

eye movement desensitization and reprocessing (EMDR):

Guided Review

1. Describe the three types of symptoms that must be present for someone to be diagnosed with PTSD.

2. What are some of the differences between PTSD and acute stress disorder?

3. How does adjustment disorder differ from PTSD?

4. Give some examples of traumatic events that tend to be associated with PTSD.

5. What sociocultural factors increase one's vulnerability to developing PTSD?

6. What aspects of the traumatic event are associated with increased risk for PTSD?

7. What psychological factors are associated with increased risk for PTSD?

8. Describe biological factors that are related to an increased risk for PTSD?

9. Describe cognitive-behavioral therapy for the treatment of PTSD.

10. Give some examples of stress management techniques for the treatment of PTSD.

11. What is EMDR, and what is known about its effectiveness for the treatment of PTSD?

12. What medications have been shown to reduce symptoms of PTSD?

13. Describe some culture-specific treatments for PTSD.

CHAPTER TEST

A. <u>Multiple Choice</u>. Choose the **best answer** to each question below.

1. All of the following are highly active during the fight-or-flight response <u>except</u> the

    A. hypothalamus.
    B. parasympathetic nervous system.
    C. sympathetic nervous system.
    D. adrenal-cortical system.

2. What is the correct order of the phases of the general adaptation syndrome?

    A. resistance → alarm → resilience → exhaustion
    B. alarm → resistance → resilience → exhaustion
    C. resistance → resilience → alarm
    D. alarm → resistance → exhaustion

3. The safety signal hypothesis asserts that

    A. knowing when a negative event will occur makes it less stressful because it is more predictable and we can prepare for it better.
    B. uncontrollable events are more stressful than controllable events.
    C. negative events are more likely than positive events to be stressful and negatively affect physical and mental health.
    D. even positive life events can be stressful and negatively affect physical and mental health.

4. The interactive model suggests that

A. psychological factors can only cause or exacerbate physical illness in people who already have a biological vulnerability to an illness, or a mild form of the illness.
B. psychological factors influence the development and progress of physical illness by affecting people's health-related behaviors.
C. physiological factors interact with cognitive and emotional functioning.
D. psychological factors influence the development and progress of physical illness by causing physiological changes that lead to or exacerbate disease.

5. Coronary heart disease (CHD) is <u>not</u>

A. more common among men than women.
B. the leading cause of death for women.
C. more common among European Americans than African Americans.
D. a condition that runs in families.

6. Essential hypertension

A. is related to genetic causes.
B. is typically due to unknown causes.
C. is unusual, occurring among fewer than 1 million people in the United States.
D. results from neurochemical deficiencies.

7. Which of the following has <u>not</u> been shown to be related to impaired immune functioning?

A. Uncontrollable stressors
B. Negative interpersonal events
C. College exams
D. Getting married

8. The DSM-IV-TR recognizes all of the following categories of sleep disorders <u>except</u>:

A. sleep disorder due to a general medical condition.
B. substance-induced sleep disorder.
C. sleep disorder due to another mental disorder.
D. sleep disorder due to stress.

9. Stimulus control therapy is used for the treatment of

A. narcolepsy.
B. sleep apnea.
C. insomnia.
D. hypersomnia.

10. Someone who experiences cataplexy would likely be diagnosed with:

A. narcolepsy.
B. sleep apnea.
C. insomnia.
D. hypersomnia.

11. Research suggests that pessimistic people

    A. are less likely to make medical visits.
    B. are more likely to die after being diagnosed with cancer than optimists.
    C. are more likely to engage in healthy behaviors.
    D. have lower blood pressure than optimists.

12. According to Friedman and Rosenman, all of the following are components of the Type A pattern except:

    A. assertiveness.
    B. easily aroused hostility.
    C. competitive achievement strivings.
    D. a sense of time urgency.

13. Which of the following is the best predictor of coronary heart disease?

    A. Impatience
    B. Competitiveness
    C. Depression
    D. Hostility

14. Which of the following statements is true?

    A. Married people tend to have more physical illnesses than unmarried people.
    B. Married men live longer than unmarried men.
    C. Marital conflict appears to have no negative effects on health.
    D. Unmarried men live longer than married men.

15. Biofeedback

    A. is a specific type of guided mastery technique.
    B. is effective for men but not for women.
    C. is no more effective at reducing headaches and pain than relaxation techniques.
    D. is more effective at reducing headaches and pain than relaxation techniques.

16. Which of the following is not required for a diagnosis of PTSD?

    A. Reexperiencing of the traumatic event.
    B. Emotional numbing and detachment.
    C. Hypervigilance and chronic arousal.

D. Persistent and uncontrollable worry.

17. Which of the following statements is <u>true</u> about acute stress disorder?

   A. It includes symptoms of emotional numbing as well as hyperarousal.
   B. It must occur within 1 week of exposure to a stressor.
   C. It lasts longer than 4 weeks.
   D. It does not include dissociative symptoms.

18. Which of the following has been found to significantly decrease PTSD symptoms and help prevent relapse?

   A. Serotonin reuptake inhibitors.
   B. Benzodiazepines.
   C. Exposure therapy.
   D. Tricyclic antidepressants.

19. Which of the following statements is <u>true</u> about treatment for PTSD?

   A. Systematic desensitization is effective for phobias but not PTSD.
   B. Repeated exposure to one's memories of the trauma significantly reduces PTSD symptoms, but does not protect against relapse.
   C. To be effective, treatment for PTSD should be focused on the trauma rather than the client's other problems, such as marital problems.
   D. Some clients are most helped by being exposed to memories of the trauma, whereas others are most helped by avoiding memories or thoughts about the trauma.

20. Which of the following is <u>not</u> a risk factor for PTSD?

   A. Low social support.
   B. Detaching from the trauma and ongoing events.
   C. Having low stress before the trauma hits.
   D. Low cortisol levels prior to the trauma.

B. <u>True-False</u>. Select T (True) or F (False) below.

1. Cortisol is considered a stress hormone.   T   F

2. T-cells are lymphocytes that kill harmful cells.   T   F

3. Sleep apnea is a breathing-related sleep disorder.   T   F

4. The hypothalamus appears to be damaged in some PTSD patients.   T   F

5. Few refugees who have located to the United States suffer from PTSD.   T   F

C. <u>Short Answer Questions</u>.

1. Describe Norman Cousins' contribution to health psychology.

2. What are three characteristics of events that contribute to their being perceived as stressful? Describe these characteristics and give some examples.

3. What is social support? Describe some of the evidence that suggests it improves health. What kinds of social support may be detrimental?

4. What are some factors that increase one's risk of developing PTSD following a trauma?

5. Describe three therapy techniques for treating the symptoms of PTSD and discuss their effectiveness.

ANSWER KEY

<u>Multiple Choice</u>
1. B
2. D
3. A
4. A
5. C
6. B
7. D
8. D
9. C
10. A
11. B
12. A
13. D
14. B
15. C
16. D
17. A
18. A
19. D
20. C

<u>True-False</u>
1. T
2. T
3. T
4. F
5. F

<u>Short Answer Questions</u>
1. See p. 172.
2. See pp. 173–174.
3. See p. 188.
4. See pp. 200–204.
5. See pp. 204–208.

Additional Readings on Chapter 6 Topics

Baum, A., & Posluszny, D. M. (1999). Health psychology: Mapping biobehavioral contributions to health and illness. Annual Review of Psychology, 50, 137-163.

Taylor, S. E., Kemeny, M. E., Reed, G. M., Bower, J. E., & Gruenewald, T. L. (2000). Psychological resources, positive illusions, and health. American Psychologist, 55, 99-109.

Taylor, S. E., Repetti, R. L., & Seeman, T. (1997). Health psychology: What is an unhealthy environment and how does it get under the skin? Annual Review of Psychology, 48, 411-447.

Chapter 7: Anxiety Disorders

LEARNING OBJECTIVES
After reading and studying this chapter, you should be able to:

1. Identify and give examples of the four types of symptoms that constitute anxiety.

2. Know the differences between adaptive fear and maladaptive anxiety.

3. Know the key features of panic disorder and the biological and psychological theories that attempt to explain it.

4. Identify the treatments available for panic disorder as well as their advantages and disadvantages.

5. Know the key features of agoraphobia.

6. Identify the four main types of specific phobias.

7. Discuss the biological and psychological theories of phobias.

8. Discuss the effective behavioral treatments for phobias.

9. Discuss the key features of generalized anxiety disorder (GAD) and the theories that attempt to explain it.

10. Identify treatments used for GAD.

11. Discuss the key features of obsessive-compulsive disorder (OCD) and explain how obsessions and compulsions are tied to one another.

12. Discuss the biological and psychological theories of OCD.

13. Identify the treatments available for OCD.

14. Describe how the anxiety disorders discussed in this chapter vary between the sexes and across cultures.

ESSENTIAL IDEAS

I. Panic disorder

       A. Panic disorder is characterized by sudden bursts of anxiety symptoms, a sense of loss of control or unreality, and the sense that one is dying.

B. Several neurotransmitters, including norepinephrine, serotonin, GABA, and CCK have been implicated in panic disorders.

C. Panic disorder runs in families, and twin studies suggest that genetics plays a role.

D. The cognitive model suggests that people with panic disorder are hypersensitive to bodily symptoms and tend to catastrophize these symptoms.

E. The vulnerability-stress model suggests that people who develop panic disorder are born with a biological predisposition to an overactive fight-or-flight response, but they don't develop the disorder unless they also tend to catastrophize their bodily symptoms.

F. Tricyclic antidepressants, selective serotonin reuptake inhibitors, and benzodiazepines can be helpful in reducing symptoms, but these symptoms tend to recur once the drugs are discontinued.

G. Cognitive-behavioral therapy has proven as useful as antidepressants in reducing panic
symptoms and more useful in preventing relapse in panic disorder.

II. Phobias

A. People with agoraphobia fear a wide variety of situations in which they might have an emergency but not be able to escape or get help. Many people with agoraphobia also suffer from panic disorder.

B. The specific phobias include animal type phobias, natural environment type phobias, situational type phobias, and blood-injection-injury type phobias.

C. People with social phobia fear social situations in which they might be embarrassed or judged by others.

D. Psychodynamic theories of phobias suggest that they represent unconscious anxiety that has been displaced. These theories have not been supported, however.

E. Behavioral theories of phobias suggest that they develop through classical conditioning and are maintained by operant conditioning. Humans may be evolutionarily prepared to develop some types of phobias more easily than others.

F. Cognitive theories have focused on social phobia and suggest that this disorder develops in people who have excessively high standards for their social performance, assume that others are judging them harshly, and are hypervigilant to signs of rejection from others.

G. Biological theories of phobias attribute their development to heredity.

H. Behavioral treatments for phobias include systematic desensitization, modeling, and flooding.

I. Cognitive techniques are used to help clients identify and challenge negative, catastrophizing thoughts they have when anxious. Group cognitive therapy has proven highly effective in the treatment of social phobia and in preventing relapse.

J. The benzodiazepines and antidepressant drugs can help to quell anxiety symptoms, but people soon relapse into phobias after the drugs have been discontinued.

III. Generalized anxiety disorder

A. Generalized anxiety disorder is characterized by chronic symptoms of anxiety across most situations.

B. Freud suggested that GAD develops when people cannot find ways to express their impulses and fear the expression of these impulses. Newer psychodynamic theories suggest that children whose parents are not sufficiently warm and nurturing develop images of the self as vulnerable and images of others as hostile, which results in chronic anxiety. Neither of these theories has been supported empirically.

C. Humanistic theory suggests that generalized anxiety results in children who develop a harsh set of self-standards they feel they must achieve in order to be acceptable.

D. Existential theory attributes generalized anxiety to existential anxiety, a universal fear of the limits and responsibilities of one's existence.

E. Cognitive theories suggest that both the conscious and unconscious thoughts of people with GAD are focused on threat.

F. Biological theories suggest that people with GAD have a deficiency in GABA or GABA receptors. They may also have a genetic predisposition to generalized anxiety.

G. Cognitive-behavioral treatments for people with GAD focus on helping them confront their negative thinking.

H. Drug therapies have included the use of benzodiazepines and a newer drug called buspirone, as well as the tricyclic antidepressants and the selective serotonin reuptake inhibitors.

IV. Obsessive-compulsive disorder

A. Obsessions are thoughts, images, ideas, or impulses that are persistent, are intrusive, and cause distress, and they commonly focus on contamination, sex, violence, and repeated doubts.

B. Compulsions are repetitive behaviors or mental acts that the individual feels he or she must perform to somehow erase his or her obsessions.

C. Biological theories of OCD speculate that areas of the brain involved in the execution of primitive patterns of behavior, such as washing rituals, may be impaired in people with OCD. These areas of the brain are rich in the neurotransmitter serotonin, and drugs that regulate serotonin have proven helpful in the treatment of OCD.

D. Psychodynamic theories of OCD suggest that the obsessions and compulsions symbolize unconscious conflict or impulses and that the proper therapy for OCD involves uncovering these unconscious thoughts. These theories have not been supported.

E. Cognitive-behavioral theories suggest that people with OCD are chronically distressed,
think in rigid and moralistic ways, judge negative thoughts as more acceptable than other people do, and feel more responsible for their thoughts and behaviors. This makes them unable to turn off the negative, intrusive thoughts that most people have occasionally.

F. Compulsive behaviors develop through operant conditioning. People are reinforced for compulsive behaviors by the fact that they reduce anxiety.

G. Effective therapies for OCD involve a combination of selective serotonin reuptake inhibitors and cognitive-behavioral therapy.

V. Social approaches to the anxiety disorders

A. Social perspectives on anxiety disorders suggest that group differences are tied to environmental pressures and to social and cultural norms.

B. Women are more prone than men to panic disorder, phobias, and generalized anxiety disorder. This tendency may be tied to women's roles in society and to gender roles.

C. The manifestation of anxiety may differ across cultures. As examples, Latino cultures have *ataque de nervios* and more chronic *nervios*, and the Japanese culture has *taijin kyofu-sho*. These difficulties may represent culturally acceptable forms of panic attacks, generalized anxiety disorder, and social phobia, respectively, or they may be true culture-bound syndromes.

KEY TERMS AND GUIDED REVIEW

Key Terms

anxiety:

neurosis:

<u>Guided Review</u>

1. Give examples of somatic, emotional, cognitive, and behavioral symptoms of anxiety.

2. Summarize the differences between adaptive fear and maladaptive anxiety.

3. Give examples of parental influences on the development of anxiety in children.

Panic Disorder

<u>Key Terms</u>

panic attacks:

panic disorder:

norepinephrine:

locus ceruleus:

limbic system:

anxiety sensitivity:

interoceptive awareness:

tricyclic antidepressants:

selective serotonin reuptake inhibitors:

benzodiazepines:

systematic desensitization:

<u>Guided Review</u>

1. What is required for someone to be diagnosed with panic disorder?

2. What are some negative ways in which panic disorder affects people's lives?

3. What is the evidence that genetics play a role in panic disorder?

4. What is the evidence that norepinephrine is involved in panic attacks?

5. What is the evidence that serotonin is involved in panic attacks?

6. How might hormones contribute to panic attacks in women?

7. Summarize the kindling model proposed by Gorman and colleagues.

8. What are some ways in which panic attacks can be induced in people with panic disorder?

9. Summarize the cognitive model of panic disorder.

10. What is the evidence that anxiety sensitivity and interoceptive awareness are important in panic disorder?

11. Describe the vulnerability-stress model of panic disorder.

12. What are the advantages and disadvantages of using tricyclic antidepressants, SSRIs, and benzodiazepines to treat panic disorder?

13. Describe some of the techniques used in cognitive-behavioral therapy for panic disorder.

14. What is the evidence that cognitive-behavioral therapy is effective in treating panic disorder?

Phobias

Key Terms

agoraphobia:

specific phobias:

animal type phobias:

natural environment type phobias:

situational type phobias:

blood-injection-injury type phobias:

social phobia:

negative reinforcement:

prepared classical conditioning:

applied tension technique:

modeling:

flooding:

Guided Review

1. What are the primary sources of anxiety for people with agoraphobia?

2. Describe the four main types of specific phobias.

3. How does social phobia differ from specific phobias?

4. How did Freud attempt to explain phobias?

5. Explain how phobias might develop through classical conditioning.

6. How can classical and operant conditioning work together to maintain a phobia?

7. What is the evidence that people are predisposed by evolution to develop certain fears?

8. How does social phobia develop, according to cognitive theories?

9. What is the evidence that genetics contribute to the development of phobias, and why is the genetic vulnerability to agoraphobia said to be sex-linked?

10. Describe some cognitive and behavioral techniques used to treat phobias.

11. What medications are used to treat phobias? Are they as effective as cognitive and behavioral therapies?

Generalized Anxiety Disorder

Key Terms

generalized anxiety disorder (GAD):

realistic anxiety:

neurotic anxiety:

moral anxiety:

conditions of worth:

existential anxiety:

automatic thoughts:

gamma-aminobutyric acid (GABA):

buspirone:

Guided Review

1. Summarize the main features of GAD. How does it differ from other anxiety disorders?

2. How did Freud attempt to explain GAD?

3. What are the humanistic and existential theories of generalized anxiety?

4. What is the evidence that maladaptive cognition contributes to GAD?

5. Why might some individuals develop a tendency to be especially vigilant to perceived threat?

6. What biological factors appear to play a role in GAD?

7. What psychological and biological treatments are effective for GAD?

Obsessive-Compulsive Disorder

Key Terms

obsessions:

compulsions:

obsessive-compulsive disorder (OCD):

caudate nucleus:

Guided Review

1. What are the symptoms of OCD?

2. How prevalent is OCD, and which groups are most likely to develop it?

3. What are some common foci of obsessions?

4. Give some examples of compulsions that are logically tied to obsessions, as well as compulsions that result from magical thinking.

5. Describe how dysfunction in brain circuitry (including the caudate nucleus) is hypothesized to be involved in OCD.

6. Summarize the psychodynamic explanation for OCD.

7. According to cognitive-behavioral theory, why do individuals with OCD have difficulty turning off intrusive thoughts?

8. According to cognitive-behavioral theory, how do compulsions develop?

9. What biological treatments are effective for OCD?

10. Describe the techniques used in cognitive-behavioral therapy for OCD.

Sociocultural Approach to the Anxiety Disorders

<u>Guided Review</u>

1. What are some reasons that more women than men may experience anxiety disorders?

2. Give an example of an anxiety-related problem that occurs in another culture.

CASE EXAMPLE
Read the following description and answer the questions below:

Stan's father died three months ago after a protracted illness. On the day of his father's funeral, Stan experienced an episode of dizziness, sweating, and had a sense that his limbs were not attached to his body. This lasted for about an hour and then disappeared. Over the next several months, however, these sensations came more frequently.

When interviewed by a therapist, Stan was tense, worried, and frightened. He sat on the edge of his chair and fidgeted constantly. He reported that for the last month, he has had a chronic sense of edginess, and an inability to maintain his concentration on anything for very long. He frequently has periods in which he feels his heart racing, he is dizzy, his ears ring, and he feels he may faint. "I think I'm going crazy!" he says. He has been thoroughly examined by his physician, and no medical causes of his symptoms can be found.

Stan's inability to concentrate interferes with his performance on the job to such an extent that his supervisor told him to get some help or he was at risk of losing his job. Stan is constantly vigilant for signs that he is having another "attack." He worries constantly about his physical and mental condition, and the possibility that he might lose his job.

1. What two anxiety disorders might Stan be suffering from, and why?

2. How would you determine which of these two diagnoses should be considered the "primary" or predominant diagnosis?

3. What is the prognosis for successful treatment of Stan's symptoms? Does it depend on which diagnosis he has?

4. What course of treatment might be most useful for Stan?

CHAPTER TEST

A. <u>Multiple Choice</u>. Choose the **best answer** to each question below.

1. Which of the following statements about panic disorder is <u>false</u>?

    A. About 40 percent of people will develop panic disorder at some time in their lives.
    B. Panic disorder tends to be chronic once it begins.
    C. About one third to one half of people with panic disorder develop agoraphobia.
    D. Panic disorder typically develops between late adolescence and the mid-30s.

2. People with panic disorder may have poorly regulated levels of _____, which is concentrated in a brain area called _____.

    A. norepinephrine; locus ceruleus
    B. serotonin; locus ceruleus
    C. epinephrine; periaqueductal gray
    D. GABA; basal ganglia

3. The kindling model of panic disorder suggests that _____ is involved in the production of panic attacks whereas _____ is involved in diffuse, anticipatory anxiety.

    A. serotonin; norepinephrine
    B. locus ceruleus; the limbic system
    C. the limbic system; locus ceruleus
    D. cholecystokinin; the periaqueductal grey

4. Which of the following statements is <u>not</u> consistent with cognitive theories of panic disorder?

    A. People with panic disorder tend to misinterpret their bodily sensations in a negative way.
    B. People with panic disorder tend to exaggerate the consequences of their symptoms.
    C. People with panic disorder tend to focus excessively on their bodily sensations.
    D. People with panic disorder tend to become angry and frustrated about their symptoms.

5. Which of the following statements about the treatment of panic disorder is true?

    A. Benzodiazepines offer the most long-lasting effects in reducing symptoms of panic disorder.
    B. The SSRIs are much more effective than the tricyclic antidepressants in reducing anxiety symptoms.
    C. The effects of cognitive-behavioral therapy are more long-lasting than the effects of antidepressants.

D. Buspirone is more effective than cognitive-behavioral therapy in reducing symptoms of panic disorder.

6. Which of the following statements about agoraphobia is <u>false</u>?

   A. To be diagnosed with agoraphobia, a person must also have panic attacks.
   B. Agoraphobia tends to develop before the age of 25.
   C. Agoraphobia tends to develop within one year after a person experiences frequent anxiety symptoms.
   D. People with agoraphobia fear both wide-open and enclosed spaces.

7. People with _____ phobia experience significant drops in heart rate and blood pressure when confronted with their feared stimulus:

   A. animal type
   B. natural environment type
   C. blood-injection-injury
   D. situational type

8. Which of the following statements is <u>false</u>?

   A. About 7 percent of people meet criteria for social phobia at some point during their lifetime.
   B. Most people who develop social phobia seek treatment for their symptoms since it is such a debilitating problem.
   C. Social phobia tends to develop during the adolescent years.
   D. Social phobia is often comorbid with antisocial personality disorder.

9. Which of the following statements is <u>false</u>?

   A. According to the safety signal hypothesis, people remember the places in which they have had panic attacks and associate these places with their symptoms.
   B. Evolution may have prepared us biologically to learn certain associations quickly, such as a fear of spiders.
   C. Phobias do not appear to be completely learned behavior: there is some evidence for a genetic contribution.
   D. According to behavioral theories, phobias develop through operant conditioning but are maintained by classical conditioning.

10. The applied tension technique is an effective treatment for:

   A. animal type phobia.
   B. natural environment type phobia.
   C. social phobia.
   D. blood-injection-injury type phobia.

11. Which of the following statements about GAD is <u>false</u>?

    A. About 4 percent of the U.S. population experiences GAD in any 6-month period.
    B. The majority of people with GAD also have another anxiety disorder.
    C. People with GAD report feeling restless most of the time and becoming tired only rarely.
    D. People with GAD tend to worry about many things instead of focusing on one issue or concern.

12. According to Freud, _____ anxiety occurs when we have been punished for expressing our id impulses.

    A. moral
    B. neurotic
    C. realistic
    D. generalized

13. Current biological theories of generalized anxiety disorder (GAD) implicate _____, which is an _____ neurotransmitter.

    A. norepinephrine; excitatory
    B. GABA; inhibitory
    C. GABA; excitatory
    D. serotonin; inhibitory

14. Biological theories of OCD propose that impulses arise in the _____ and are carried to the _____.

    A. caudate nucleus; thalamus
    B. orbital frontal cortex; caudate nucleus
    C. thalmus; orbital frontal cortex
    D. orbital frontal cortex; hypothalamus

15. Which of the following is <u>not</u> a reason why people with OCD have trouble turning off their negative thoughts?

    A. People with OCD may have a tendency toward rigid, moralistic thinking.
    B. People with OCD are often depressed or anxious much of the time.
    C. People with OCD equate having negative thoughts with actually engaging in the behaviors.
    D. People with OCD do not believe they should be able to control their thoughts.

16. A neurotransmitter involved in the production of OCD symptoms and which, when treated, leads to improvement in symptoms, is:

A. Norepinephrine.
B. GABA.
C. Epinephrine.
D. Serotonin.

17. The most common focus of obsessive thoughts is

A. sexual impulses.
B. aggressive impulses.
C. dirt and contamination.
D. repeated doubts.

18. The failure of which type of drug to treat OCD effectively provided a clue that OCD was different from the other anxiety disorders?

A. Serotonin reuptake inhibitors.
B. Tricyclic antidepressants.
C. Benzodiazepines.
D. Barbiturates.

19. Which of the following theories has not been proposed to explain gender differences in anxiety disorders?

A. Women are believed to produce fewer of the neurochemicals that reduce anxiety as compared to men.
B. Men are socialized to confront feared situations and, thus, conquer their anxiety.
C. Men may self-medicate with alcohol rather than seek treatment for anxiety symptoms.
D. Due to women's lack of power in society, they tend to have stronger feelings of vulnerability and defenselessness.

20. Which of the following is not a characteristic of *ataque de nervios*?

A. Falling to the ground and convulsing.
B. Becoming unable to speak.
C. Difficulty breathing.
D. Difficulty moving limbs.

B. True-False. Select T (True) or F (False) below.

1. The parents of anxious children tend to be controlling and overprotective.   T   F

2. Interoceptive awareness refers to a heightened awareness of bodily sensations that resemble the beginning sensations of a panic attack.   T   F

3. Claustrophobia is an example of a social phobia.   T   F

4. Existential anxiety develops when we are repeatedly prevented from expressing our id impulses.　　T　　F

5. In OCD, compulsions are always logically tied to an individual's specific obsessions (e.g., obsessions about contamination lead people to wash their hands).　　T　　F

C. Short Answer Questions.

1. What are the advantages and disadvantages of prescribing medications for people with panic disorder?

2. Describe two theories (one biological, one psychological) of panic disorder. What evidence supports each theory?

3. Describe how phobias develop and are maintained, according to behavioral theories?

4. Use a vulnerability-stress model to explain how an individual might develop generalized anxiety disorder.

5. Describe the cognitive-behavioral treatment of OCD and discuss its effectiveness.

ANSWER KEY

Case Example
1. Panic disorder: episodes of dizziness, sweating, sense of limbs not attached to body, heart racing, thoughts of going crazy, worries about future attacks; generalized anxiety disorder: chronic symptoms of tension, worry, edginess, problems in concentrating that interfere with his job.
2. If Stan's anxiety is primarily about having a panic attack, then panic disorder is the primary diagnosis. If his anxiety is about a number of events and activities, then generalized anxiety disorder is a more appropriate diagnosis.
3. The prognosis for the successful treatment of panic disorder is quite good; for generalized anxiety disorder it is not as good.

4. Cognitive-behavioral treatments have been effective in treating symptoms like Stan's. Antidepressant drugs can also be helpful.

Multiple Choice
1. A
2. A
3. B
4. D
5. C
6. A
7. C
8. B
9. D
10. D
11. C
12. A
13. B
14. B
15. D
16. D
17. C
18. C
19. A
20. B

True-False
1. T
2. T
3. F
4. F
5. T

Short Answer Questions
1. See pp. 227–228.
2. See pp. 223–227.
3. See pp. 238–239.
4. See pp. 245–249, 261.
5. See p. 258.

Additional Readings on Chapter 6 Topics
        Bouton, M. E., Mineka, S., & Barlow, D. H. (2001). A modern learning theory perspective on the etiology of panic disorder. Psychological Review, 108, 4-32.
        Shoenberger, D. (2002). Discontinuing paroxetine (Paxil): A personal account. Psychotherapy and Psychosomatics, 71, 237-238.

Wells, A. (2002). Worry, metacognition, and GAD: Nature, consequences, and treatment. <u>Journal of Cognitive Psychotherapy, 16,</u> 179-192.

Chapter 8: Somatoform and Dissociative Disorders

LEARNING OBJECTIVES
After reading and studying this chapter, you should be able to:

1. Distinguish among somatoform disorders, psychosomatic disorders, malingering, and factitious disorders.

2. Define conversion disorder and la belle indifference, and discuss how early physicians and psychodynamic theorists viewed it.

3. Discuss the types of traumas frequently experienced by people with conversion disorder, and the other disorders that often accompany it.

4. Describe the psychodynamic and behavioral treatments for conversion disorder.

5. Distinguish among somatization disorder, pain disorder, conversion disorder, and hypochondriasis.

6. Discuss the cultural and cohort variations in the rates of somatization disorder, as well as the disorders that often accompany it and those that are similar to it, making it difficult to diagnose.

7. Discuss the possible causes of somatization disorder.

8. Summarize how clinicians conduct psychotherapy for people with somatization disorder.

9. Define body dysmorphic disorder, and describe the behaviors that people with this disorder engage in to compensate for their "defective" body part(s).

10. Describe conditions that are related to body dysmorphic disorder and how they have influenced the treatment of this disorder.

11. Discuss how early theorists such as Freud viewed dissociation, how Hilgard's experiments provided insight into the "hidden observer" phenomenon, and how these views have shaped our modern understanding of dissociative disorders.

12. Identify the symptoms of dissociative identity disorder (DID) and the different types of alternate personalities that people with DID may exhibit.

13. Identify correlates of DID, including risk factors and comorbid conditions.

14. Describe the theories of DID and the different approaches to treating it.

15. Define dissociative fugue, and explain how it is similar to and different from other dissociative disorders.

16. Discuss the conditions that may precede a dissociative fugue.

17. Distinguish among anterograde, retrograde, organic, and psychogenic amnesia, and know the types of information that tend to be lost and retained in each type.

18. Define depersonalization disorder.

19. Discuss the controversy surrounding the issue of repressed memories.

ESSENTIAL IDEAS

I. Somatoform disorders

    A. Somatoform disorders are a group of disorders in which people experience significant physical symptoms for which there is no apparent organic cause.

    B. Conversion disorder involves loss of functioning in a part of the body for no organic reason. Conversion symptoms often occur after trauma or stress, perhaps because the person cannot face memories or emotions associated with the trauma. Treatment for conversion disorder focuses on expression of emotions or memories associated with the symptoms.

    C. Somatization disorder involves a long history of multiple physical complaints for which people have sought treatment but for which there is no apparent organic cause. Pain disorder involves only the experience of chronic, unexplainable pain. These disorders appear to be common, particularly among women, young children, the elderly, and people of Asian or Hispanic heritage.

    D. Hypochondriasis is a condition in which people worry chronically about having a dread disease, despite evidence that they do not. This disorder appears to be rare.

    E. In somatization disorder, pain disorder, and hypochondriasis, individuals often have a history of anxiety and depression. These disorders may represent acceptable ways of expressing emotional pain.

    F. Cognitive theories of the disorders say that they are due to excessive focus on physical symptoms and the tendency to catastrophize symptoms. Treatment for these disorders involves helping people to identify the feelings and thoughts behind the symptoms and to find more adaptive ways of coping.

    G. People with body dysmorphic disorder have an obsessional preoccupation with some parts of their bodies and make elaborate attempts to change these body parts. Treatments for body dysmorphic disorder include psychodynamic therapy to reveal underlying concerns, systematic desensitization therapy to reduce obsessions and compulsions about the body, and selective serotonin reuptake inhibitors.

II. Dissociative disorders

A. The dissociative disorders include dissociative identity disorder (DID), dissociative fugue, dissociative amnesia, and depersonalization disorder.

B. In all these disorders, people's conscious experiences of themselves become fragmented, they may lack awareness of core aspects of themselves, and they may experience amnesia for important events.

C. The distinct feature of dissociative identity disorder is the development of multiple separate personalities within the same person. The personalities take turns being in control.

D. People with dissociative fugue move away from home and assume entirely new identities, with complete amnesia for their previous identities. They do not switch back and forth between different personalities.

E. People with dissociative amnesia lose important memories due to psychological causes.

F. People with depersonalization disorder have frequent experiences of feeling detached from their mental processes or their bodies.

G. These disorders are often, although not always, associated with traumatic experiences.

H. Therapists often treat these disorders by helping people explore past experiences and feelings that they have blocked from consciousness and by supporting them as they develop more integrated experiences of self and more adaptive ways of coping with stress.

I. Significant controversy exists over the validity of the diagnoses of dissociative disorders and the notion of repressed memories.

KEY TERMS AND GUIDED REVIEW

Key Terms

dissociation:

Somatoform Disorders

Key Terms

somatoform disorders:

psychosomatic disorders:

malingering:

factitious disorders:

factitious disorder by proxy:

conversion disorder:

la belle indifference:

glove anesthesia:

somatization disorder:

pain disorder:

hypochondriasis:

body dysmorphic disorder:

<u>Guided Review</u>

1. What is the difference between somatoform disorders and psychosomatic disorders?

2. How do somatoform disorders differ from malingering and factitious disorders?

3. Describe the features of conversion disorder and conditions often associated with it.

4. How can we tell conversion disorder apart from a physical disorder?

5. Describe how you would treat someone with a conversion disorder.

6. What are the symptoms of somatization disorder and how does it differ from pain disorder?

7. What are some ways in which clinicians attempt to distinguish between somatization and actual symptoms of physical illnesses?

8. How do the rates of somatization disorder vary by age, culture, and gender?

9. What do family history and twin studies suggest about the heritability of somatization and pain disorder?

10. Describe the cognitive theory of somatization and pain disorder.

11. What is the relationship between trauma and somatization and pain disorder?

12. Describe some approaches used to treat somatization and pain disorder.

13. What are some similarities and differences between somatization and hypochondriasis?

14. Describe the features of body dysmorphic disorder including gender differences in focus on specific body parts.

14. What are some of the other conditions that are related to body dysmorphic disorder?

15. Describe some approaches used to treat body dysmorphic disorder.

CASE EXAMPLE
Read the following description and answer the questions below:

Betty has belonged to the health maintenance organization funded by her health insurance for only three years, but already her medical records fill three large binders. Betty is convinced that she has serious heart disease. She can describe many times when she has had "painful feelings" in her upper chest. When she has these feelings, she stops everything, lies quietly for a long time, and listens to her heart. She reports that her heart "races and pounds" and that there are frequent irregularities in her heart beat. Numerous medical tests, including two occasions when her heart was monitored for a 24-hour period, have revealed no irregularities or abnormalities in her heart beat. Now she is insisting that she should have a cardiac catheterization, an invasive medical procedure that her physicians think is totally unnecessary.

Heart disease is only the latest ailment that Betty is convinced she has. For several years, she has believed she has a kidney disease. She carefully monitors the color of her urine and the frequency of her urination. She has these data charted in a diary she keeps of her health. In her diary, she also lists any pains or twinges she has each day. Betty spends a lot of time researching possible causes of her pains on computer databases. When she goes to her physician, at least once a month, she takes along her diary and her notes on the diseases they may indicate. Betty insists on going over each of these entries in her diary, one at a time, with her physician. Over the last three years, in addition to her cardiac tests, she has undergone many X-rays, an MRI scan, multiple ultrasound tests, and almost monthly blood and urine tests (she usually brings in a sample of her urine to her physician when she visits). None of these tests has ever indicated any disease.

1. Which of the somatoform disorders is the most appropriate diagnosis for Betty? How did you, or would you, rule out any of the other somatoform disorders?

2. What family or developmental history might have led Betty to have the concerns she exhibits?

3. How is Betty likely to respond to a recommendation that she needs to see a psychiatrist instead of a cardiologist?

4. What treatment would you prescribe for Betty?

Dissociative Disorders

<u>Key Terms</u>

dissociative identity disorder (DID):

dissociative fugue:

dissociative amnesia:

organic amnesia:

anterograde amnesia:

psychogenic amnesia:

retrograde amnesia:

depersonalization disorder:

<u>Guided Review</u>

1. What are some common dissociative experiences and possible causes of these experiences?

2. What is the hidden observer phenomenon, and what is the evidence that it exists?

3. Describe some of the gender differences in DID.

4. What are the symptoms of DID?

5. Describe the common types of alters.

6. Describe some ways in which children tend to manifest DID.

7. What are some reasons for the increasing number of DID diagnoses?

8. What are some theories of how DID develops?

9. Describe some techniques used to treat DID.

10. What are some characteristics of people who experience dissociative fugues?

11. What is the difference between organic and psychogenic amnesia?

12. What is the difference between anterograde and retrograde amnesia?

13. Describe some of the explanations for psychogenic amnesias.

14. What is the repressed memory debate? Describe the views on both sides of this debate.

CHAPTER TEST

A. <u>Multiple Choice</u>. Choose the **best answer** to each question below.

1. In the somatoform disorders, the physical symptoms

    A. are caused by organic factors, but are made worse by the somatoform disorder.
    B. are consciously produced by the person with the disorder.
    C. are deliberately faked to get attention from medical providers.
    D. remit when the psychological factors producing them are treated.

2. People who worry chronically that they have a physical disease in the absence of evidence that they do and who frequently seek medical attention would be diagnosed with

    A. conversion disorder.
    B. pain disorder.
    C. body dysmorphic disorder.
    D. hypochondriasis.

3. Body dysmorphic disorder involves

    A. a history of complaints about pain that appears to have no physical cause.
    B. excessive preoccupation with some part of the body the person believes is defective.
    C. loss of functioning in some part of the body for psychological rather than physical reasons.
    D. chronic worry that one has a physical disease in the absence of evidence that one does.

4. Someone who fakes a symptom or disorder to avoid some unwanted situation would be regarded as

    A. having a factitious disorder by proxy.
    B. having a psychosomatic disorder.
    C. malingering.
    D. having somatization disorder.

5. Someone with a factitious disorder

    A. deliberately fakes an illness to avoid an unwanted situation.

B. deliberately fakes an illness to gain medical attention.

C. experiences psychological stress in the form of physical symptoms.

D. has psychological factors that negatively influence an actual physical illness.

6. Sigmund Freud found that when people tended to recall painful memories or emotions that they had blocked from consciousness, usually under hypnosis

A. they experienced relief from glove anesthesia.

B. they experienced relief from la belle indifference.

C. they developed symptoms of DID.

D. they realized that their physical symptoms had psychological causes.

7. To be diagnosed with somatization disorder, a person must have all of the following except:

A. two gastrointestinal symptoms.

B. a history of taking numerous medications for physical symptoms.

C. one sexual symptom.

D. no organic causes of their physical complaints.

8. People with somatization disorder are more likely to

A. be Caucasian.

B. be male.

C. be older in age.

D. have a history of sexual abuse.

9. Body dysmorphic disorder is thought by some researchers to be a form of

A. generalized anxiety disorder.

B. schizophrenia.

C. somatization disorder.

D. obsessive-compulsive disorder.

10. Which of the following interventions is typically not used to treat body dysmorphic disorder?

A. Hypnosis

B. SSRIs

C. Preventing compulsive behaviors related to body parts

D. Challenging distorted thoughts about the body

11. A process in which different parts of an individual's identity, memories, or consciousness become split off from one another is known as

A. somatization.

B. dissociation.

C. psychogenic amnesia.

D. la belle indifference.

12. Which of the following is <u>not</u> a common type of alter in DID?

    A. Helper personality
    B. Persecutor personality
    C. Intellectual alter
    D. Child alter

13. Which of the following statements about children with DID is <u>false</u>?

    A. Children with DID tend to exhibit antisocial behavior.
    B. Children with DID tend to show symptoms of posttraumatic stress disorder.
    C. Children with DID tend to hear voices inside their heads.
    D. Children with DID tend to experience delusions and hallucinations.

14. Most people with DID do <u>not</u>

    A. also meet criteria for major depression.
    B. have a history of being physically abused.
    C. tend to be stubborn and resistant to suggestion.
    D. tend to have significant periods of amnesia.

15. Cross-cultural research has found that _____ are more likely to experience dissociative symptoms than other ethnic groups.

    A. Latinos
    B. African Americans
    C. Caucasians
    D. Asian Americans

16. Which of the following statements about DID is <u>false</u>?

    A. DID is diagnosed more often in the U.S. than in Europe.
    B. DID is believed to be primarily caused by dysregulation of norepinephrine.
    C. The diagnostic criteria for DID first appeared in DSM-III, which was published in 1980.
    D. Most people diagnosed with DID are also diagnosed with a personality disorder.

17. In _____, people cannot remember important facts about their lives and their personal identities, but are aware that there are large gaps in their memories.

    A. dissociative identity disorder
    B. dissociative fugue
    C. depersonalization disorder

D. dissociative amnesia

18. The inability to remember new information is known as

    A. retrograde amnesia.
    B. psychogenic amnesia.
    C. anterograde amnesia.
    D. dissociative amnesia.

19. Between 25–40 percent of people arrested for homicide claim to have _____.

    A. amnesia
    B. DID
    C. conversion disorder
    D. depersonalization disorder

20. Which of the following experiences is relatively common, occurring in approximately half of all adults at some time during their life?

    A. Depersonalization
    B. Fugue
    C. Self-mutilation
    D. Glove anesthesia

B. True-False. Select T (True) or F (False) below.

1. About 90 percent of patients with DID have a history of suicide attempts.   T   F

2. DID is more commonly diagnosed in the U.S. than in Europe, but body dysmorphic disorder is more often diagnosed in Europe than the U.S.   T   F

3. People with somatoform disorders do not consciously fake their symptoms, but people with psychosomatic disorders do fake their symptoms.   T   F

4. Korsakoff's syndrome is an example of a somatoform disorder.   T   F

5. Body dysmorphic disorder is more common among younger adults, whereas somatization disorder is more common among older adults.   T   F

C. Short Answer Questions.

1. Describe how you would attempt to distinguish between conversion disorder and actual physical ailments.

2. How is a dissociative fugue different from dissociative amnesia?

3. Provide some arguments for and against the existence of repressed memories.

4. Distinguish between hypochondriasis and somatization disorder.

5. How are somatoform disorders different from psychosomatic disorders, malingering, and factitious disorders?

ANSWER KEY

Case Example
1. Hypochondriasis; ruled out somatization disorder because she does not have the variety of complaints necessary for somatization disorder.
2. Having a family member die of heart disease or kidney disease; having a family member who modeled hypochondriasis; having been reinforced by attention from others for her physical complaints.
3. Not well because she truly believes she is ill.
4. Help Betty find more adaptive ways of coping with the stresses in her life and of gaining attention from others; help her confront the irrationality of her medical concerns.

Multiple Choice
1. D
2. D
3. B
4. C
5. B
6. A
7. B
8. C
9. D
10. A
11. B
12. C
13. D
14. C
15. A
16. B
17. D
18. C
19. A
20. A

True-False
1. F
2. T
3. F
4. F
5. T

Short Answer Questions
1. See pp. 273–274.
2. See pp. 290–292.

3. See pp. 294–295.
4. See pp. 274–279.
5. See pp. 269–270.

Additional Readings on Chapter 8 Topics

Lilienfeld, S. O., Kirsch, I., Sarbin, T. R., Lynn, S. J., Chaves, J. F., Ganaway, G. K., & Powell, R. A. (1999). Dissociative identity disorder and the sociocognitive model: Recalling the lessons of the past. Psychological Bulletin, 125, 507-523.

Merckelbach, H., Devilly, G. J., & Rassin, E. (2002). Alters in dissociative identity disorder: Metaphors or genuine entities? Clinical Psychology Review, 22, 481-498.

Phillips, K. A. (2000). Body dysmorphic disorder: Diagnostic controversies and treatment challenges. Bulletin of the Menninger Clinic, 64, 18-35.

Chapter 9: Mood Disorders

LEARNING OBJECTIVES
After reading and studying this chapter, you should be able to:

1. Distinguish between unipolar and bipolar depression, and know the diagnostic criteria for the disorders that fall under each category: major depression (and its associated subtypes), dysthymic disorder, double depression, bipolar I disorder, bipolar II disorder, cyclothymic disorder, and rapid cycling bipolar disorder.

2. Explain how depression affects the whole person, i.e., cognitively, emotionally, behaviorally, and physiologically.

3. Discuss how rates of unipolar depression vary as a function of age, gender, and culture, as well as the proposed explanations for these differences.

4. Summarize the evidence for the idea that bipolar disorder is linked to creativity.

5. Summarize the evidence for and against the idea that genetics partially determine who will develop a mood disorder.

6. Discuss the monoamine theory of depression.

7. Discuss the neuroendocrine and neurophysiological abnormalities in depression.

8. Discuss research on the relationship between depression and hormone levels in women.

9. Discuss the behavioral, psychodynamic, learned helplessness, reformulated learned helplessness, cognitive, ruminative response styles, and interpersonal theories of depression.

10. Describe how social values and social status impact the experience of depression.

11. Discuss how tricyclic antidepressants, monoamine oxidase inhibitors, and selective serotonin reuptake inhibitors work, their side effects, and their effectiveness for treating depression.

12. Discuss the type of patient most likely to receive electroconvulsive therapy (ECT), what the therapy entails, and how it might work.

13. Discuss how repetitive transcranial magnetic stimulation (rTMS) and vagus nerve stimulation (VNS) work and their effectiveness for treating depression.

14. Explain how light therapy for seasonal affective disorder might work.

15. Discuss drugs used to treat bipolar disorder and describe their side effects.

16. Describe behavior, cognitive-behavioral, interpersonal, and psychodynamic therapies for the treatment of depression.

17. Compare the effectiveness of cognitive-behavioral, interpersonal, and drug therapies for the treatment of depression.

18. Discuss how depression may be successfully prevented.

ESSENTIAL IDEAS

I. Unipolar depression

A. Depression includes disturbances in emotion (sadness, loss of interest), bodily function (loss of sleep, appetite, and sexual drive), behavior (retardation or agitation), and thought (worthlessness, guilt, suicidality).

B. The two primary categories of unipolar depressive disorders are major depression and dysthymic disorder. There are several subtypes of major depression.

C. Young adults have the highest rates of depression.

D. Many people who become depressed remain so for several months or more and have multiple relapses over their lifetimes.

II. Bipolar Disorder

A. The symptoms of mania include elation, irritation and agitation, grandiosity, impulsivity, and racing thoughts and speech. People with bipolar disorder experience periods of both mania and depression.

B. The two major diagnostic categories of bipolar mood disorders are bipolar disorder and cyclothymic disorder.

C. Bipolar mood disorders are less common than depressive disorders, but they are equally common in men and women.

D. The onset of bipolar disorders is most often in late adolescence or early adulthood. Most people with bipolar disorder have multiple episodes.

E. There is some evidence that people with mood disorders are more creative.

III. Biological theories of mood disorders

A. Genetic factors clearly play a role in bipolar disorder, although it is somewhat less clear what role genetics play in many forms of unipolar depression.

B. The neurotransmitter theories suggest that imbalances in levels of norepinephrine or serotonin or the dysregulation of receptors for these neurotransmitters contributes to depression, and dysregulation of norepinephrine, serotonin, or dopamine is involved in bipolar disorder.

C. Neuroimaging studies have shown abnormalities in the structure and functioning of the prefrontal cortex, hippocampus, anterior cingulate cortex, and amygdala in people with mood disorders.

D. People with depression have chronic hyperactivity of the hypothalamic-pituitary-adrenal axis, which helps to regulate the body's response to stress.

E. Abnormalities in the biological stress response may result from early stressors in some people and contribute to depression.

IV. Psychological theories of mood disorders

A. The behavioral theories of depression suggest that stress can induce depression by reducing the number of reinforcers available to people.

B. The learned helplessness theory of depression says that uncontrollable events can lead people to believe that important outcomes are outside of their control and thus can lead them to develop depression.

C. The cognitive theories of depression argue that people with depression think in distorted and negative ways, and this leads them to become depressed, particularly in the face of negative events. In addition, people who ruminate about their depressive symptoms and the causes and consequences of those symptoms appear more prone to develop severe levels of depression.

D. Psychodynamic theories posit that people with depression are overly dependent on the evaluations and approval of others for their self-esteem, as a result of poor nurturing by parents.

E. The interpersonal theories of depression suggest that poor attachment relationships early in life can lead children to develop expectations that they must be or do certain things in order to win the approval of others, which puts them at risk for depression. They may also engage in excessive reassurance-seeking, which drives away their social support.

V. Social perspectives on mood disorders

A. More recent generations appear to be at higher risk for depression than earlier generations, perhaps because of historical changes in values and social structures related to depression.

B. People of lower social status tend to have higher rates of depression. Women's greater vulnerability to depression may be tied to their lower social status and the risks of abuse that accompany this social status.

C. Less industrialized cultures may have lower rates of depression than more industrialized cultures. Some studies suggest that the manifestation of depression and mania may be different across cultures.

VI. Mood disorders treatments

A. Tricyclic antidepressants are effective in treating depression but have some side effects and can be dangerous in overdose.

B. The monoamine oxidase inhibitors (MAOIs) also are effective treatments for depression but can interact with certain medications and foods.

C. The selective serotonin reuptake inhibitors (SSRIs) are effective treatments for depression and have become popular because they are less dangerous and their side effects are more tolerable than are those of other drug treatments.

D. Electroconvulsive therapy (ECT) involves inducing seizures in people with depression. It can be quite effective but is controversial.

E. Lithium is useful in the treatment of mood disorders but requires careful monitoring to prevent dangerous side effects.

F. Anticonvulsants, antipsychotics, and calcium channel blockers can also help to relieve mania.

G. Behavioral treatment focuses on increasing positive reinforcers and decreasing aversive events by helping clients change their environments, learn social skills, and learn mood-management skills.

H. Cognitive-behavioral treatment combines the techniques of behavior therapy with techniques to identify and challenge depressive thinking patterns.

I. Psychodynamic therapy focuses on uncovering unconscious hostility and fears of abandonment through the interpretation of transference, memories, and dreams.

J. Interpersonal therapy seeks to identify and overcome problems with grief, role transitions, interpersonal role disputes, and deficits in interpersonal skills that contribute to depression.

K. Cognitive-behavioral therapy, interpersonal therapy, and drug treatments seem to work equally well with the majority of people with depression, and the combination of drug therapy and one of these psychotherapies may be the most effective.

L. Some research suggests that interventions targeting high risk groups can help to prevent or delay first onsets of depression.

KEY TERMS AND GUIDED REVIEW

<u>Key Terms</u>

bipolar disorder:

mania:

depression:

unipolar depression:

<u>Guided Review</u>

1. What is the difference between unipolar and bipolar depression?

Unipolar Depression

<u>Key Terms</u>

delusions:

hallucinations:

major depression:

dysthymic disorder:

double depression:

seasonal affective disorder (SAD):

<u>Guided Review</u>

1. What are the emotional, behavioral, physiological, and cognitive symptoms of depression?

2. What are the differences between major depression and dysthymic disorder?

3. Describe the subtypes of depression.

4. Discuss how the prevalence of depression varies with age and why it might vary.

5. Describe the course of depression and how treatment is believed to affect the course.

6. What are some of the long-term effects of depression among both children and adults?

7. How does puberty affect boys and girls differently with respect to depression?

Bipolar Disorder

<u>Key Terms</u>

bipolar I disorder:

bipolar II disorder:

hypomania:

cyclothymic disorder:

rapid cycling bipolar disorder:

<u>Guided Review</u>

1. What are the symptoms of mania?

2. What are the differences between bipolar I disorder, bipolar II disorder, and cyclothymic disorder?

3. How common in bipolar disorder? What are some of its long-term effects?

4. What are some ways in which creativity and bipolar disorder may be related?

Biological Theories of Mood Disorders

<u>Key Terms</u>

monoamines:

norepinephrine:

serotonin:

dopamine:

monoamine theories:

hypothalamic-pituitary-adrenal (HPA) axis:

cortisol:

premenstrual dysphoric disorder:

<u>Guided Review</u>

1. What is the evidence that mood disorders have a genetic basis?

2. What neurotransmitter abnormalities appear to be present in unipolar and bipolar depression?

3. Describe the brain abnormalities associated with depression. What might be causing these brain abnormalities?

4. What is the HPA axis, and how is it altered in depression?

5. What is the evidence that women's hormones are related to depression?

6. What is the evidence that early traumatic stress is related to a vulnerability to depression?

Psychological Theories of Mood Disorders

<u>Key Terms</u>

behavioral theory of depression:

learned helplessness theory:

learned helplessness deficits:

negative cognitive triad:

reformulated learned helplessness theory:

causal attribution:

depressive realism:

ruminative response styles theory:

rumination:

introjected hostility:

interpersonal theories of depression:

contingencies of self-worth:

excessive reassurance seeking:

<u>Guided Review</u>

1. Describe Lewinsohn's behavioral theory of depression.

2. What is learned helplessness theory and what evidence supports it?

3. Describe Beck's cognitive theory of depression.

4. What is the reformulated learned helplessness theory and what evidence supports it?

5. What is depressive realism, and how does it refute the idea that individuals with depression suffer from errors in thinking?

6. What is rumination, and what are the effects of rumination on mood? How is rumination related to gender?

7. According to psychodynamic theory, what leads to depression?

8. Describe the interpersonal theory of depression.

Sociocultural Perspectives on Mood Disorders

<u>Key Terms</u>

cohort effect:

<u>Guided Review</u>

1. What is a cohort effect and how might such an effect account for age differences in depression?

2. What are the relationships among social status, gender, and depression?

3. Give some examples of how depression may differ across cultures.

Mood Disorders Treatments

<u>Key Terms</u>

tricyclic antidepressant drugs:

monoamine oxidase inhibitors (MAOIs):

selective serotonin reuptake inhibitors (SSRIs):

electroconvulsive therapy (ECT):

repetitive transcranial magnetic stimulation (rTMS):

vagus nerve stimulation (VNS):

light therapy:

lithium:

anticonvulsants:

antipsychotic drugs:

calcium channel blockers:

behavior therapy:

cognitive-behavioral therapy:

interpersonal therapy (IPT):

psychodynamic therapy:

Guided Review

1. How effective are tricyclic antidepressants and MAOIs for treating depression? What are some of the side effects of these drugs?

2. Describe some of the advantages that SSRIs have over other antidepressant medications?

3. What are some of the side effects of SSRIs?

4. What are some of the advantages of bupropion? What are some of the side effects associated with this drug?

5. For whom is ECT prescribed? How effective is ECT, and what are some reasons why it remains controversial?

6. What is rTMS, and how does it work?

7. How does VNS appear to decrease depressive symptoms?

6. How does light therapy for SAD appear to work?

7. How effective is lithium for bipolar disorder? What are some side effects and/or difficulties associated with taking it?

8. Other than lithium, what are some drugs used to treat bipolar disorder?

9. Describe some of the strategies used in behavior therapy for depression.

10. Describe some of the techniques used in cognitive-behavioral therapy for depression.

11. Describe how interpersonal therapy for depression is conducted. How is it similar to and different from cognitive-behavioral therapy?

12. Describe some of the techniques used in psychodynamic therapy to treat depression.

13. How do psychotherapies and drug therapies compare in effectiveness?

14. Describe an intervention designed to prevent depression.

CASE EXAMPLE
Read the following description and answer the questions below:

Amanda is a successful businesswoman, who apparently has everything going for her. She has plenty of money, a nice car, a good network of friends. Yet she is quite depressed. This depression seems to have been chronic for the past three years. Amanda feels down most of the time, although when good things happen she can feel some pleasure. Amanda says she is chronically tired and drained, like her whole body is weighted down. In part because she stopped exercising when she began feeling depressed, Amanda has gained 30 pounds in the last three years. Despite her success, her self-esteem is low and she frequently makes berating comments about herself and the future. Amanda clearly has continued to function at a rather high level -- at least most of the time. A couple of times in the last three years, however, Amanda has had periods in which her depressive symptoms become much more severe and she cannot function at all. These periods tend to last about a month. Then they pass, but Amanda always returns to her chronic moderately depressed level, rather than ever really feeling good.

1. List all of the specific symptoms of depression that Amanda shows.

2. What diagnosis (or diagnoses) fits Amanda's symptoms? Specify the symptoms that lead you to this diagnosis.

3. What kinds of information about Amanda would (a) an interpersonal therapist, and (b) a cognitive-behavioral therapist want to know in order to plan a course of treatment for her?

CHAPTER TEST

A. Multiple Choice. Choose the **best answer** to each question below.

1. A person who has experienced (for the past month) a loss of interest in his or her usual activities, in addition to psychomotor agitation, increased appetite, insomnia, and thoughts of committing suicide, would be diagnosed as having

    A. double depression.
    B. biplolar II disorder.
    C. major depression.
    D. cyclothymic disorder.

2. Someone who experiences a loss of interest in his or her usual activities, as well as psychomotor retardation hypersomnia, and loss of energy for more than two years, would be diagnosed as having

    A. dysthymic disorder.
    B. major depression.
    C. double depression.
    D. cyclothymic disorder.

3. With which subtype of depression would the person in the following case example be diagnosed?
    Laura, a 30-year-old graduate student, has always been a "sensitive person." She feels happy at times, but generally feels low. She has been eating more lately and has gained weight. She has also been sleeping a lot lately.

    A. Depression with catatonic features
    B. Depression with melancholic features
    C. Depression with psychotic features
    D. Depression with atypical features

4. The lowest rates of depression are found among people

    A. over 85 years old.
    B. between 15 and 24 years of age.
    C. younger than 15 years.
    D. between 55 and 70 years of age.

5. During adolescence:

    A. rates of depression increase among boys but stay the same among girls.
    B. rates of depression increase among girls but stay the same among boys.

C. rates of depression increase among both boys and girls.
D. rates of depression decrease for both boys and girls.

6. A person who alternates between episodes of hypomania and moderate depression chronically for at least two years would be diagnosed as having

   A. bipolar I disorder.
   B. bipolar II disorder.
   C. rapid cycling bipolar disorder.
   D. cyclothymic disorder.

7. Andre has a history of severe depression, but recently experienced symptoms of rapid speech, racing thoughts, and significant irritation and agitation that lasted for two weeks. During this time, he did not sleep for several days. What diagnosis best fits Andre's experience?

   A. Bipolar I disorder
   B. Bipolar II disorder
   C. Cyclothymic disorder
   D. Major depression

8. Evidence that there is a relationship between bipolar disorder and creativity comes largely from

   A. psychodynamic theory.
   B. analysis of brain structures.
   C. family studies.
   D. cognitive theories.

9. Which of the following statements is <u>false</u> about the role of genetics in mood disorders?

   A. Family history studies have found that the first-degree relatives of people with bipolar disorder are 2-3 times more likely to have either bipolar or unipolar depression.
   B. Family history studies have found that the first-degree relatives of people with unipolar depression are more likely than controls to have either bipolar or unipolar depression.
   C. Twin studies have yielded more equivocal results for unipolar depression than for bipolar depression.
   D. Fewer than 10 percent of the first-degree relatives of people with bipolar disorder will develop the disorder themselves.

10. All of the following neurotransmitters have been implicated in unipolar depression <u>except</u>:

   A. glutamate.
   B. norepinephrine.
   C. serotonin.
   D. dopamine.

11. A brain area that appears to be overactive in depressed people is the

    A. cerebellum.
    B. cerebral cortex.
    C. HPA axis.
    D. anterior cingulate.

12. All of the following increase a woman's risk of developing postpartum depression <u>except</u>:

    A. hormonal imbalances.
    B. a past history of depression.
    C. having a fussy baby.
    D. lack of social support.

13. The idea that life stress leads to depression by causing a reduction in positive reinforcers is known as

    A. learned helplessness theory.
    B. reformulated learned helplessness theory.
    C. depressive realism.
    D. Lewinsohn's behavioral theory.

14. The <u>reformulated</u> learned helplessness theory added which of the following notions to learned helplessness theory?

    A. The negative cognitive triad
    B. Rumination
    C. Depressive realism
    D. Causal attributions

15. Freud's introjected hostility theory of depression suggests that

    A. individuals become depressed when their contingencies of self-worth are not met.
    B. depression develops when individuals feel abandoned and turn their anger inward.
    C. individuals who are depressed are modeling the sadness and anger they observed in early caregivers.
    D. depression results from insecure attachments during childhood.

16. _____ have potentially serious side effects, such as dangerous interactions with over-the-counter medications and the amino acid tyramine.

    A. Tricyclic antidepressants
    B. SSRIs
    C. MAOIs
    D. Calcium channel blockers

17. Which of the following statements about ECT is <u>false</u>?

        A. ECT is typically administered bilaterally.
        B. Modern ECT does not cause significant memory problems.
        C. ECT is administered more often in midwestern and eastern states.
        D. About 85 percent of patients relapse into depression after receiving ECT.

18. Which of the following statements about lithium is <u>false</u>?

        A. Lithium is more effective at reducing symptoms of mania than symptoms of depression.
        B. Lithium causes the side effect tardive dyskinesia.
        C. Lithium has been shown to reduce relapses of mania.
        D. Lithium can be toxic if taken in too high a dose.

19. A functional analysis in behavior therapy focuses on

        A. identifying an individual's overall level of functioning in the community.
        B. identifying the circumstances that lead to a person's depressive symptoms.
        C. helping an individual identify their negative thinking patterns.
        D. evaluating an individual's level of self-worth.

20. Regarding treatment effectiveness, research has found that

        A. drug therapies are more effective at reducing symptoms of depression than psychological treatments.
        B. interpersonal therapy is the most effective intervention for treating depression.
        C. cognitive-behavioral therapy and drug therapies are equally effective in reducing depression.
        D. combining psychotherapy with medication offers no increased benefit to patients than receiving either treatment alone.

B. <u>True-False</u>. Select T (True) or F (False) below.

1. Vagus nerve stimulation involves repeated electric shock to the brain.   T   F

2. Approximately half of women who experience childbirth will develop postpartum depression.   T   F

3. Girls who mature earlier than their peers tend to have higher rates of depression than girls who mature later.   T   F

4. Rapid cycling bipolar disorder is characterized by having four or more cycles of mania and depression within a year.   T   F

5. Women are more prone than men to both unipolar and bipolar depression.　　T　　F

C. Short Answer Questions.

1. Contrast cognitive theories of depression with the notion of "depressive realism." Can both theories be accurate? Why or why not?

2. Do women's hormones play a role in their higher rates of depression? Cite evidence from the chapter to support your argument.

3. Describe how ECT is administered. Who is most likely to benefit from it? What are some of the shortcomings of ECT?

4. Describe some of the cognitive-behavioral techniques used to treat depression.

5. What are some of the brain abnormalities that occur in depression?

ANSWER KEY

Case Example
1. Depressed mood, chronic fatigue, heavy laden feeling in body, weight gain, low self-esteem, hopelessness.
2. Dysthymic disorder with atypical features (chronic depressed mood, low self-esteem, hopelessness, but ability to experience pleasure, weight gain, heavy feelings in body), and double depression (symptoms sometimes become much worse and severely interfere with functioning, but she returns only to dysthymia).
3. A cognitive-behavioral therapist would want to know specifically what "berating comments" Amanda tends to make about herself and the future and what thoughts Amanda has during those times when she feels most down. CB therapist would also want to know how Amanda views her success and her friends and whether she discounts all the good things in her life. An interpersonal therapist would want to know more about Amanda's circle of friends and the quality of those friendships, any recent losses Amanda perceives in her life, whether Amanda is

experiencing any role conflicts or role transitions, and the strength of Amanda's interpersonal skills.

Multiple Choice
1. C
2. A
3. D
4. D
5. B
6. D
7. A
8. C
9. B
10. A
11. C
12. A
13. D
14. D
15. B
16. C
17. A
18. A
19. B
20. C

<u>True-False</u>
1. F
2. F
3. T
4. T
5. F

<u>Short Answer Questions</u>
1. See pp. 321–323.
2. See pp. 317–319.
3. See pp. 332–334.
4. See pp. 338–340.
5. See pp. 315–317.

<u>Additional Readings on Chapter 9 Topics</u>

Ferguson, J. M. (2001). The effects of antidepressants on sexual functioning in depressed patients: A review. <u>Journal of Clinical Psychiatry, 62 Suppl 3,</u> 22-34.

Jacobson, N. S., Dobson, K. S., Truax, P. A., Addis, M. E., Koerner, K., Gollan, J. K., Gortner, E., & Prince, S. E. (1996). A component analysis of cognitive-behavioral treatment for depression. <u>Journal of Consulting and Clinical Psychology, 64,</u> 295-304.

Teasdale, J. D., Moore, R. G., Hayhurst, H., Pope, M., Williams, S., & Segal, Z. V. (2002). Metacognitive awareness and prevention of relapse in depression: Empirical evidence. <u>Journal of Consulting and Clinical Psychology, 70,</u> 275-287.

Chapter 10: Suicide

LEARNING OBJECTIVES

After reading and studying this chapter, you should be able to:

1. Identify Shneidman's types of people who commit suicide.

2. Discuss suicide rates and how they vary by gender, ethnicity, nationality, and age.

3. Discuss the sociocultural, psychological, and biological theories of suicide.

4. Identify reasons why it is difficult to study suicide scientifically.

5. Discuss Durkheim's sociological theory of suicide.

6. Discuss suicide contagion and why it might occur.

7. Discuss the mental disorders associated with suicide.

8. Describe the biological, psychological, and sociocultural interventions for suicide.

9. Discuss the relationship between guns and suicide.

10. Identify and explain the major arguments in the current debate concerning whether people should have the right to commit suicide.

11. Integrate the various factors contributing to suicide according to a diathesis-stress model.

ESSENTIAL IDEAS

I. Defining and measuring suicide

      A. Suicide is defined as death from injury, poisoning, or suffocation when there is evidence (either explicit or implicit) that the injury was self-inflicted and that the decedent intended to kill himself or herself.

      B. Death seekers clearly and explicitly seek to end their lives. Death initiators also have a clear intention to die but believe that they are simply hastening an inevitable death. Death ignorers intend to end their lives but do not believe this means the end of their existence. Death darers are ambivalent about dying and take actions that greatly increase their chances of death but that do not guarantee they will die.

      C. Suicide is the eighth leading cause of death in the United States. Internationally, at least 160,000 people die by suicide and an additional 2 million people make suicide attempts each year.

D. Women are more likely than men to attempt suicide, but men are more likely than women to complete suicide.

E. Cross-cultural differences in suicide rates may have to do with religious doctrines, stressors, and cultural norms about suicide.

F. Young people are less likely than adults to commit suicide, but suicide rates have been rising dramatically for young people in recent decades. The elderly, particularly elderly men, are at high risk for suicide.

II. Understanding suicide

A. Suicide notes suggest that mental anguish and escape from pain are behind many suicides.

B. Several negative life events or circumstances increase risk for suicide, including economic hardship, serious illness, loss, and abuse.

C. Durkheim distinguished among egoistic suicide, which is committed by people who feel alienated from others, empty of social contacts, and alone in an unsupportive world; anomic suicide, which is committed by people who experience severe disorientation because of a major change in their relationships to society; and altruistic suicide, which is committed by people who believe that taking their own lives will benefit society in some way.

D. Suicide clusters occur when two or more suicides or attempted suicides are nonrandomly bunched in space or time. This phenomenon is sometimes called suicide contagion.

E. Psychodynamic theorists attribute suicide to repressed rage, which leads to self-destruction.

F. Several mental disorders increase risk for suicide, including depression, bipolar disorder, substance abuse, schizophrenia, and anxiety disorders.

G. Cognitive-behavioral theorists argue that hopelessness and dichotomous thinking contribute to suicide.

H. Impulsivity is a behavioral characteristic common to many people who commit suicide.

I. Family history, twin, and adoption studies all suggest there is a genetic vulnerability to suicide.

J. Many studies have found a link between low serotonin levels and suicide.

III. Treatment and prevention

      A. Drug treatments for suicidality most often involve lithium or antidepressant medications to reduce impulsive and violent behavior, depression, and mania. Antipsychotic medications and other medications that treat the symptoms of an existing mental disorder may also be used.

      B. Psychotherapies for suicide are similar to those used for depression. Dialectical behavior therapy has been specifically designed to address skills deficits and thinking patterns in people who are suicidal.

      C. Suicide hot lines and crisis intervention programs provide immediate help to people who are highly suicidal.

      D. Community prevention programs aim to educate the public about suicide and encourage suicidal people to enter treatment.

      E. Guns are involved in the majority of suicides, and some research suggests that restricting access to guns can reduce the number of suicide attempts.

      F. Society is debating whether people have a right to choose to commit suicide.

KEY TERMS AND GUIDED REVIEW

Defining and Measuring Suicide

<u>Key Terms</u>

suicide:

death seekers:

death initiators:

death ignorers:

death darers:

subintentional deaths:

<u>Guided Review</u>

1. Explain what this sentence means: "Suicide-like behaviors fall on a continuum."

2. Describe the similarities and differences among death seekers, death initiators, death ignorers, and death darers.

3. What are some reasons why it is difficult to obtain accurate suicide rates?

4. How does one's gender affect one's likelihood of attempting or completing suicide?

5. How do suicide rates vary by ethnicity?

6. Discuss the suicide rate among children and adolescents. What are some of the risk factors for suicide in this age group?

7. What contributes to suicide among the elderly?

Understanding Suicide

<u>Key Terms</u>

egoistic suicide:

anomic suicide:

altruistic suicide:

suicide cluster:

suicide contagion:

impulsivity:

hopelessness:

dichotomous thinking:

<u>Guided Review</u>

1. Describe some of the barriers to research on suicide.

2. What are some sociocultural factors that appear to increase one's risk of suicide?

3. Describe Durkheim's three types of suicide.

4. What is a suicide cluster? What are some contributors to suicide clusters?

5. Summarize Freud's theory of suicide.

6. What is the evidence that mental disorders are associated with suicide?

7. What are some cognitive and behavioral contributors to suicide?

8. What is the evidence that suicide has a genetic basis?

9. What is the evidence that serotonin is related to suicide?

Treatment and Prevention

<u>Key Terms</u>

crisis intervention:

suicide hot lines:

dialectical behavior therapy:

euthanasia:

<u>Guided Review</u>

1. Describe some community-based programs for suicide.

2. What are some medications that may be prescribed to prevent suicide?

3. What psychotherapies may be used to prevent suicide?

4. What are some advantages and disadvantages of sociocultural interventions for suicide?

5. What is the relationship between guns and suicide?

6. Describe gender differences in euthanasia.

CASE EXAMPLE
Read the following description and answer the questions below:

Brian was fed up and couldn't take it anymore. He had been depressed for quite a while and was living with some people in a house rampant with drug use in a crime-ridden area. Freaks and gangsters would frequently stop by and "hang out." This was not the life Brian had envisioned for himself. In high school, he had been a bright and popular guy, often the object of many girls' affections. He was a brilliant artist and musician, and had spent a year at a prestigious art college in Chicago living out his fantasies. However, Brian had been using drugs for several years and had been engaging in risky, impulsive actions at school. He and a friend would ride the subway and spray-paint graffiti on city walls late at night. These excursions would take them into areas rife with crime.

Brian began to develop a feeling of emptiness and he could not explain to himself how he had gotten so far off track. His girlfriend broke up with him and he lost his job. He wondered if he was gay. His roommates were starting to steal his money and his musical equipment. Some of them were getting involved in gangs. Brian abruptly left one day for Chicago, where for a time he had known peace, but got a speeding ticket on the way. This was too much for him. He taped a suicide note to a highway sign and pulled his car onto a deserted road. With his painting supplies in the back seat, it did not take long for Brian to die once he set his car ablaze while sitting behind the wheel.

1. Which one of Shneidman's types of people who commit suicide is Brian?

2. What are some of the warning signs that suggest Brian may be at risk for suicide?

3. Which one of Durkheim's types of suicides is this case?

CHAPTER TEST

A. <u>Multiple Choice</u>. Choose the **best answer** to each question below.

1. Suicide is the _____ leading cause of death in the United States.

    A. second
    B. fifth
    C. eighth
    D. twelfth

2. Which of the following is <u>not</u> part of the CDC's definition of suicide?

    A. There is evidence that the injury was self-inflicted.
    B. There is evidence that the person was depressed or unhappy.
    C. There is evidence that the person intended to kill himself or herself.
    D. Suicide is death from injury, poisoning, or suffocation.

3. Death initiators

    A. clearly and explicitly seek to end their lives.
    B. intend to end their lives but do not believe this means the end of their existence.
    C. have a clear intention to die, but believe they are simply hastening an inevitable death.
    D. are ambivalent about dying, and take actions that greatly increase their chances of death, but do not guarantee that they will die.

4. Death ignorers

A. clearly and explicitly seek to end their lives.
B. intend to end their lives but do not believe this means the end of their existence.
C. have a clear intention to die, but believe they are simply hastening an inevitable death.
D. are ambivalent about dying, and take actions that greatly increase their chances of death, but do not guarantee that they will die.

5. According to Shneidman, which of the following terms would apply to someone with skin cancer who continues to frequent tanning booths?

A. Subintentional death
B. Death ignorer
C. Death darer
D. Death seeker

6. Women are _____ likely than men to attempt suicide. Men are _____ likely than women to complete suicide.

A. three times more; two times less
B. two times more; four times more
C. three times more; four times more
D. four times more; three times less

7. Men are more likely than women to do all of the following except:

A. take a drug overdose.
B. shoot themselves.
C. stab themselves.
D. drink alcohol when they are distressed.

8. Which ethnic group has the highest suicide rate in the U.S.?

A. Native Americans
B. African Americans
C. Asians
D. Whites

9. Which of the following nations has the highest suicide rate (among the nations listed)?

A. Mexico
B. United States
C. Australia
D. England

10. All of the following are risk factors for suicide in adolescents except:

A. aggressive behavior.

B. obesity.
C. a suicide attempt by a friend.
D. increased drug and alcohol use.

11. The single best predictor of future suicide attempts and completions is

A. drug and alcohol abuse.
B. ownership of a handgun.
C. impulsivity.
D. a previous history of a suicide attempt.

12. Which of the following statements about barriers to understanding suicide is <u>false</u>?

A. Suicide is a rare event.
B. Family members and friends may selectively remember information about the victim.
C. The majority of people who contemplate suicide never complete it.
D. The majority of suicide completers leave suicide notes.

13. Suicide committed by people who experience severe disorientation because of a large change in their relationships with society is known as

A. altruistic suicide.
B. egoistic suicide.
C. anomic suicide.
D. pessimistic suicide.

14. Suicide committed by people who feel alienated from others, empty of social contacts, and alone in an unsupportive world is known as

A. altruistic suicide.
B. egoistic suicide.
C. anomic suicide.
D. pessimistic suicide.

15. One problem with Freud's theory of suicide is that

A. it claims that suicidal people are depressed, but most suicidal people suffer from schizophrenia.
B. people do not tend to express anger in suicide notes because they cannot express these emotions and are turning the feelings in on themselves.
C. suicidal people tend to direct their anger at the part of their ego that represents a lost love object.
D. it is difficult to test and therefore hard to evaluate.

16. The most common disorder among people who commit suicide is

A. schizophrenia.
B. anorexia nervosa.
C. depression.
D. substance abuse.

17. Which of the following is <u>not</u> a common characteristic of suicidal individuals?

A. Anger and rage
B. Guilt and despair
C. Hopelessness
D. Dichotomous thinking

18. Which of the following statements is <u>false</u>?

A. Ten to fifteen percent of people with schizophrenia commit suicide.
B. Depression increases one's risk of suicide, but mania does not.
C. Individuals who are impulsive and also have a mental disorder are at increased risk for attempting suicide.
D. As many as 10 percent of people who complete suicide would not have met criteria for a diagnosable mental disorder.

19. All of the following increase one's risk of suicide <u>except</u>

A. hopelessness.
B. a family history of suicidality.
C. dichotomous thinking.
D. excessively high serotonin levels.

20. The medication(s) most consistently shown to reduce risk of suicide is/are

A. SSRIs.
B. antipsychotics.
C. lithium.
D. MAOIs.

B. <u>True-False</u>. Select T (True) or F (False) below.

1. Approximately 10 percent of college students report attempting suicide while at college.
   T   F

2. Research has shown that suicide does not run in families.   T   F

3. Recent studies have found SSRIs to increase the risk of suicide in some individuals.
   T   F

4. Suicide rates decrease when cities or states limit people's access to guns.   T   F

5. The rates of suicide have increased for children and adolescents in recent years, but have declined for the elderly.   T   F

C. <u>Short Answer Questions</u>.

1. Describe some of the risk factors for suicide.

2. What are some interventions that may help reduce or prevent suicide?

3. How do the rates of suicide vary by gender, age, and ethnicity?

4. Describe several stressful life events that appear to contribute to suicide risk.

5. What are some reasons why it is difficult to study suicide?

ANSWER KEY

Case Example
1. A death darer.
2. Male gender, drug use, between the ages of 15 and 24, social withdrawal, recent loss, impulsivity.
3. Anomic suicide.

Multiple Choice
1. C
2. B
3. C
4. B
5. A
6. C
7. A
8. D
9. C
10. B
11. D
12. D
13. C
14. B
15. D
16. C
17. A
18. B
19. D
20. C

True-False
1. T
2. T
3. T
4. T
5. T

Short Answer Questions
1. See pp. 360–367.
2. See pp. 367–370.
3. See pp. 355–359.
4. See pp. 361–363.
5. See pp. 354–355.

Additional Reading on Chapter 10 Topics

Gould, M. S., & Kramer, R. A. (2001). Youth suicide prevention. <u>Suicide and Life-Threatening Behavior, 31,</u> 6-31.

Sanchez, H. G. (2001). Risk factor model for suicide assessment and intervention. <u>Professional Psychology: Research and Practice, 32,</u> 351-358.

Tondo, L., Ghiani, C., & Albert, M. (2001). Pharmacologic interventions in suicide prevention. <u>Journal of Clinical Psychiatry, 62,</u> 51-55.

Chapter 11: Schizophrenia

LEARNING OBJECTIVES

After reading and studying this chapter, you should be able to:

1. Describe the prevalence of schizophrenia and how it varies by gender and ethnicity.

2. Define and describe delusions and hallucinations, as well as the different types of delusions and hallucinations, and how they vary and do not vary across cultures.

3. Describe the disorganized thought and speech that occurs with schizophrenia.

4. Distinguish between disorganized and catatonic behavior.

5. Describe common negative symptoms of schizophrenia.

6. Discuss the history of diagnostic criteria for schizophrenia, as well as the current criteria for schizophrenia and disorders that are similar to it.

7. Distinguish between Type I and Type II symptoms, as well as between prodromal and residual symptoms.

8. Identify the key features of each of the five subtypes of schizophrenia: paranoid, disorganized, catatonic, undifferentiated, and residual.

9. Describe the prognosis for an individual with schizophrenia and how it might vary according to the gender and age of the affected individual.

10. Discuss the evidence for a genetic transmission of schizophrenia, and which people are most at risk for developing schizophrenia.

11. Discuss the brain areas implicated in schizophrenia, as well as their functions, and be able to discuss how they are different in the brains of people with schizophrenia compared to people without schizophrenia.

12. Discuss both past and recent hypotheses of how dopamine is believed to affect the development and treatment of schizophrenia.

13. Discuss the psychosocial factors associated with schizophrenia and the evidence for them.

14. Discuss the drug therapies most commonly prescribed for schizophrenia, their side effects, which symptoms they treat most effectively, and which ones they do not.

15. Discuss the psychological and social interventions designed for people with schizophrenia.

ESSENTIAL IDEAS

I. Symptoms, diagnosis, and course

A. The positive, or Type I, symptoms of schizophrenia are delusions, hallucinations, disorganized thinking and speech, and disorganized or catatonic behavior. The forms of delusions and hallucinations are relatively similar across cultures, but the specific content varies by culture.

B. The negative, or Type II, symptoms are affective flattening, poverty of speech, and loss of motivation.

C. Other symptoms of schizophrenia include anhedonia, inappropriate affect, and impaired social skills.

D. Prodromal symptoms are more moderate positive and negative symptoms that are present before an individual goes into an acute phase of the illness, and residual symptoms are symptoms present after an acute phase.

E. The DSM-IV-TR differentiates between schizophrenia and two other disorders that include severe mood symptoms. In mood disorders with psychotic features, the mood symptoms occur in the absence of the schizophrenic symptoms at least some of the time. In schizoaffective disorder, the schizophrenic symptoms occur in the absence of the mood symptoms.

F. The DSM-IV-TR further differentiates among paranoid, disorganized, catatonic, undifferentiated, and residual schizophrenia.

II. Biological theories

A. There is strong evidence for a genetic contribution to schizophrenia, although genetics do not fully explain who has the disorder.

B. Many people with schizophrenia show significant structural and functional abnormalities in the brain, including low frontal activity and enlarged ventricles.

C. A number of prenatal and birth difficulties are implicated in the development of schizophrenia, including prenatal hypoxia and exposure to the influenza virus during the second trimester of gestation.

D. Difficulties in deploying attention may be at the core of many symptoms of schizophrenia.

E. Excess dopamine activity in the mesolimbic pathway, and unusually low dopamine activity in the prefrontal area of the brain, may work together to create the symptoms of schizophrenia.

F. New research suggests that serotonin, glutamate, and GABA may also play a role in schizophrenia.

III. Psychosocial perspectives

A. People with schizophrenia tend to live in highly stressful circumstances. Most theorists see this as a consequence, rather than as a cause of, schizophrenia.

B. Early psychodynamic theories viewed schizophrenia as the result of harsh and inconsistent parenting, which caused an individual to regress to infantile forms of coping. According to other theories, families put schizophrenic members in double binds or have deviant patterns of communication. These theories have not been supported.

C. Families high in expressed emotion are overinvolved and overprotective while being critical and resentful. People with schizophrenia who live in families high in expressed emotion may be at increased risk for relapse.

D. Behavioral theorists view schizophrenic behaviors as the result of operant conditioning.

E. Cognitive theorists see some schizophrenic symptoms as attempts to understand perceptual and attentional disturbances.

F. Different cultures have different native theories of schizophrenia.

IV. Treatments

A. The phenothiazines were the first drugs to have a significant effect on schizophrenia. They are more effective in treating the positive symptoms than the negative symptoms, however, and a significant percentage of people do not respond to them at all. They can induce a number of serious side effects, including tardive dyskinesia.

B. New drugs, called atypical antipsychotics, seem more effective in treating schizophrenia than the phenothiazines and have fewer side effects.

C. Psychosocial therapies focus on helping people with schizophrenia and their families to understand and cope with the consequences of the disorder. They also help the person with schizophrenia gain resources and integrate into the community to the extent possible.

D. Studies show that providing psychosocial therapy along with medication can significantly reduce the rate of relapse in schizophrenia.

E. Community-based comprehensive treatment programs for people with schizophrenia have been underfunded. As a result, many people with this disorder receive little or no useful treatment.

F. Traditional healers treat people with schizophrenia within the context of their cultural beliefs.

KEY TERMS AND GUIDED REVIEW

<u>Key Terms</u>

psychosis:

schizophrenia:

<u>Guided Review</u>

1. How common is schizophrenia, and where do many people with schizophrenia reside?

2. How do the rates of schizophrenia vary by gender and ethnicity?

Symptoms, Diagnosis, and Course

<u>Key Terms</u>

positive symptoms:

negative symptoms:

delusions:

persecutory delusion:

delusion of reference:

grandiose delusions:

delusions of thought insertion:

hallucinations:

auditory hallucination:

visual hallucination:

tactile hallucinations:

somatic hallucinations:

formal thought disorder:

word salad:

smooth pursuit eye movement:

working memory:

catatonia:

catatonic excitement:

affective flattening:

alogia:

avolition:

dementia praecox:

prodromal symptoms:

residual symptoms:

paranoid schizophrenia:

disorganized schizophrenia:

catatonic schizophrenia:

echolalia:

echopraxia:

undifferentiated schizophrenia:

residual schizophrenia:

Guided Review

1. Give some examples of positive and negative symptoms in schizophrenia.

2. How do delusions differ from self-deceptions?

3. Describe some different types of delusions.

4. How do delusions differ across cultures?

5. Describe some different types of hallucinations.

6. How do hallucinations differ across cultures?

7. Describe the speech and thought abnormalities in schizophrenia.

8. Describe some deficits in cognition and attention that many people with schizophrenia experience.

9. Describe the behavioral abnormalities exhibited by individuals with schizophrenia.

10. Describe some ways in which affect is exhibited in schizophrenia.

11. Why are negative symptoms difficult to diagnose reliably?

12. Summarize how the diagnostic criteria for schizophrenia have changed since the disorder was first conceptualized.

13. What is the difference between prodromal and residual symptoms?

14. What is the difference between Type I and Type II schizophrenia?

15. Describe the five types of schizophrenia.

16. How does schizophrenia vary by age and gender?

17. How do sociocultural factors contribute to schizophrenia?

Biological Theories

Key Terms

enlarged ventricles:

prefrontal cortex:

perinatal hypoxia:

dopamine:

phenothiazines (neuroleptics):

mesolimbic pathway:

Guided Review

1. Summarize the evidence for a genetic contribution to schizophrenia.

2. What are some of the brain areas that exhibit abnormal structure or function in schizophrenia? Which ones appear to contribute to positive symptoms, and which ones appear to contribute to negative symptoms?

3. What appear to be some of the causes of neuroanatomical abnormalities in schizophrenia?

4. What is the evidence that prenatal and birth difficulties are related to the development of schizophrenia?

5. What was the original dopamine theory of schizophrenia? Give some examples of evidence that supported it.

6. What were some of the observations that called the original dopamine theory into question?

7. How does dopamine appear to be related to schizophrenia, according to modern views?

Psychosocial Perspectives

Key Terms

social selection:

expressed emotion:

Guided Review

1. What appears to be the relationship between social selection and schizophrenia?

2. What appears to be the relationship between stress and schizophrenia?

3. Describe the early psychodynamic theories of schizophrenia.

4. Describe some family interaction and communication patterns that can contribute to or exacerbate schizophrenia.

5. Describe Beck and Rector's cognitive model of schizophrenia.

6. Describe a behavioral theory of schizophrenia.

Treatments

Key Terms

chlorpromazine:

akinesia:

akathesis:

tardive dyskinesia:

atypical antipsychotics:

agranulocytosis:

assertive community treatment programs:

Guided Review

1. Describe some of the earlier treatments for schizophrenia.

2. What symptoms do phenothiazines help reduce? How do they work?

3. Describe some of the side effects of neuroleptics.

4. How do the atypical antipsychotics differ from the neuroleptics? What are some of the most effective atypical antipsychotics, and how do they work in the brain?

5. Give examples of cognitive, behavioral, and social interventions for schizophrenia.

6. Describe some of the components of family therapy for schizophrenia.

7. Describe some of the community-level interventions for schizophrenia. What is the evidence that they are effective?

8. Identify and describe the models that traditional healers tend to follow in treating schizophrenic symptoms.

CASE EXAMPLE

Read the following description and answer the questions below:

A 29-year-old single Afro-Caribbean woman was admitted to the accident and emergency department with heavy bleeding from a laceration to the right labia majora, self-inflicted with a razor blade. She explained that she wanted to cut off her clitoris, because it was the center of her problems. She believed that her genitalia had enlarged due to masturbation and were becoming more masculine, and that this would prevent her from finding a partner and marrying.

She claimed to recall that when she was 6 years old two men had put a curse on her because of petty jealousy. She believed that they started to follow her when she turned 17, and 'made' her 'touch herself.' From age 20 she could hear the voice of a male stranger 'guiding' her, commenting on her actions and on the size of her genitals. She felt that articles on female sexuality in women's magazines were specifically directed at her. Occasionally she felt that the direction in which she walked was controlled from outside. Her family reported that from 19 years of age she had become increasingly withdrawn and that in the past six months, she had become even more preoccupied, checking her genital size each time she showered. She found it hard to concentrate at work, felt extremely self-conscious, believing that people could tell that she was abnormal. She became depressed and frequently thought of cutting off her genitalia.

There were seven siblings in the family, of which she was the fourth. She lived with her mother, her parents having divorced, and discipline appeared to be lax. An older brother had been treated for schizophrenia and there was a history of possible schizophrenia in a paternal uncle and aunt.

When she was in her early teens, her schoolwork deteriorated and she ran away frequently. At 14 she was arrested and charged for shoplifting. She left school at 15 with no close friends or qualifications, eventually obtaining work as a catering assistant, a job she held for six years.

At age 17 she started masturbating to heterosexual fantasies. She felt guilty about this, and sometimes experienced the act as being forced from outside. Despite never having seen another woman's external genitalia pictorially or in reality, she believed her own labia were grossly abnormal, and could not be reassured by advice of doctors to the contrary. There was no other psychiatric history or relevant medical history, and no drug or alcohol abuse. Physical examination was normal apart from the wound to her genitalia.

During the mental state examination, she was alert and oriented, polite and appropriate in manner,but her affect was blunted and rapport was difficult. Her mood was mildly depressed. There was poverty of speech, and some loosening of associations. Her thought content was dominated by her genital size, and she entertained ideas of further mutilation attempts, but not of suicide. She did not think she was ill and only reluctantly accepted hospitalization.

Computerized tomography (CT) showed enlargement of the frontal horn of the left lateral ventricle of her brain. (Adapted from Krasucki, Kemp, & David, 1995.)

1. Carefully read the description of the woman in the case example. What evidence could you cite that would indicate to you whether she is simply self-deceived or delusional?

2. What types of symptoms does she exhibit that suggest a particular diagnosis? Which of the schizophrenias would you diagnose her with, and why?

3. Given her condition as described in the case study, as well as her family characteristics and personal background, briefly describe your prognosis for her condition. What facts about her culture and gender suggest a particular prognosis for her, compared to someone with different characteristics?

CHAPTER TEST

A. <u>Multiple Choice</u>. Choose the **best answer** to each question below.

1. Which group is more likely to be misdiagnosed with schizophrenia?

     A. Asian Americans
     B. Hispanic Americans
     C. European Americans
     D. African Americans

2. Compared to men with schizophrenia, women with schizophrenia

     A. tend to develop schizophrenia earlier in life, particularly during their late teens or early 20s.
     B. are more likely to be married.
     C. are less likely to have had children.
     D. are less likely to have graduated from high school or college.

3. A man who believes he is Napoleon is suffering from a

     A. persecutory delusion.
     B. delusion of thought control.
     C. grandiose delusion.
     D. delusion of reference.

4. The most common type of hallucination is

     A. auditory.
     B. visual.
     C. somatic.
     D. tactile.

5. Associations between words that are based on the sounds of the words rather than the content

are known as

    A. neologisms.
    B. clangs.
    C. perseverations.
    D. word salad.

6. Individuals with schizophrenia have difficulties with

    A. working memory.
    B. distinguishing tastes.
    C. long-term memory.
    D. arithmetic.

7. Poverty of speech (reduced speaking) is known as

    A. avolition.
    B. word salad.
    C. alogia.
    D. anhedonia.

8. All of the following are negative symptoms of schizophrenia except:

    A. avolition.
    B. alogia.
    C. affective flattening.
    D. auditory hallucinations.

9. Emil Kraepelin believed that the disorder he coined _____ resulted from premature deterioration of the brain.

    A. schizophrenia
    B. format thought disorder
    C. dementia praecox
    D. multiple personality disorder

10. A person who exhibits delusions and hallucinations for 2 weeks, but who also experiences a major depressive episode following this 2-week period while continuing to experience delusions and hallucinations, would be diagnosed with

    A. schizophreniform disorder.
    B. schizoaffective disorder.
    C. shared psychotic disorder.
    D. schizophrenia.

11. Someone who speaks in word salads and does not bathe, dress, or eat if left alone, would

most likely be diagnosed with

    A. paranoid schizophrenia.
    B. catatonic schizophrenia.
    C. undifferentiated schizophrenia.
    D. disorganized schizophrenia.

12. Repetitive imitation of the movements of another person is known as

    A. catalepsy.
    B. catatonia.
    C. echolalia.
    D. echopraxia.

13. Compared to men with schizophrenia, women with the disorder

    A. tend to have more severe language impairments.
    B. tend to develop schizophrenia at an earlier age.
    C. are hospitalized less often.
    D. more often have enlarged ventricles.

14. A brain area that is important in language, emotional expression, and planning, and which is smaller and shows less activity in people with schizophrenia, is the

    A. basal ganglia.
    B. hippocampus.
    C. prefrontal cortex.
    D. temporal lobe.

15. A newer theory of dopamine and schizophrenia suggests that there is excess dopaminergic activity in the _____, but unusually low dopaminergic activity in the _____.

    A. limbic system; prefrontal area
    B. mesolimbic system; prefrontal area
    C. prefrontal area; limbic system
    D. thalamus; mesolimbic system

16. Julie's son Winston just fell down and hurt himself. She rushes to comfort him and takes him into her arms, saying, "You stupid little boy! Watch where you walk!" This is an example of

    A. a double bind.
    B. a negative symptom.
    C. communication deviance.
    D. expressed emotion.

17. Families high in expressed emotion

   A. Are both overprotective and rejecting of the schizophrenic family member, not letting him or her develop an autonomous sense of self.
   B. Express their thoughts in vague, indefinite ways and communicate misperceptions and misinterpretations.
   C. Are overinvolved with each other, are overprotective of the schizophrenic family member, and are critical and resentful of the schizophrenic family member.
   D. Tend to express their emotions when they should keep them to themselves to avoid hurting the schizophrenic family member's feelings.

18. A common side effect of phenothiazines that consists of agitation which causes patients to pace and be unable to sit still is

   A. akathesis.
   B. agranulocytosis.
   C. tardive dyskinesia.
   D. akinesia.

19. A treatment for schizophrenia that binds to the D4 dopamine receptor and influences positive as well as negative symptoms of schizophrenia is known as

   A. fish oil.
   B. thorazine.
   C. chlorpromazine.
   D. clozapine.

20. The _____ model suggests that individuals' symptoms can be reduced if they have faith in a traditional healer.

   A. social support
   B. clinical
   C. structural
   D. persuasive

B. True-False. Select T (True) or F (False) below.

1. Individuals with schizophrenia living in developing countries have a better prognosis for recovery than do individuals with schizophrenia in developed countries.   T   F

2. Delusions and hallucinations are Type II symptoms of schizophrenia.   T   F

3. Compared to other forms of schizophrenia, people with the paranoid subtype show better cognitive and emotional functioning and are more likely to hold down a job.   T   F

4. The earlier the age of onset, the more favorable the course of schizophrenia.   T   F

5. Evidence of lower activity in and/or atrophy of the prefrontal cortex is found more commonly in people with predominantly positive symptoms of schizophrenia. T   F

C. Short Answer Questions.

1. What is the relationship between dopamine and schizophrenia? Cite evidence to support your answer.

2. Do psychological factors influence schizophrenia? If so, how? Be specific.

3. Describe the five subtypes of schizophrenia.

4. Describe some ways in which the symptoms of schizophrenia may vary across cultures.

5. Based upon what you read in the chapter, describe the "ideal treatment package" for schizophrenia.

ANSWER KEY

Case Example
1. The woman is delusional, and not simply self-deceived, because she not only occasionally entertains distorted thoughts about her clitoris, but she is preoccupied with them and takes action based upon them.
2. The woman exhibits delusions of reference, hallucinations, poverty of speech, magical thinking, and loosening of associations. Her symptoms suggest a diagnosis of paranoid schizophrenia because her delusions and hallucinations center around themes of persecution and paranoia.
3. Though the woman appears to have acute symptoms, her prognosis appears somewhat favorable because paranoid schizophrenia has the best prognosis in general. However, she evidences ventricular enlargement and has a family history of schizophrenia, which suggest strong biological underpinnings and brain atrophy, which make her prognosis less favorable. She shows evidence of being able to hold down a consistent job, which is favorable. Her lack of social support is unfavorable, as is the early onset of her symptoms. However, the course of schizophrenia tends to be more favorable for women. Her residence in a developed country (England) is not favorable for her prognosis.

Multiple Choice
1. D
2. B
3. C
4. A
5. B
6. A
7. C
8. D
9. C
10. B
11. D
12. D
13. C
14. C
15. B
16. A
17. C
18. A
19. D
20. B

True-False

1. T
2. F
3. T
4. F
5. F

Short Answer Questions

1. See pp. 399–400.
2. See pp. 403–406.
3. See pp. 391–392.
4. See pp. 384–385.
5. A good answer would include biological, psychological, and social components to the treatment package as described in the chapter (e.g., clozapine, individual and family therapy).

Additional Reading on Chapter 11 Topics

Evans, J. D., Heaton, R. K., Paulsen, J. S., McAdams, L. A., Heaton, S. C., Jeste, D. V. (1999). Schizoaffective disorder: A form of schizophrenia or affective disorder? Journal of Clinical Psychiatry, 60, 874-882.

Pilling, S., Bebbington, P., Kuipers, E., Garety, P., Geddes, J., Orbach, G., & Morgan, C. (2002). Psychological treatments in schizophrenia: I. Meta-analysis of family intervention and cognitive behaviour therapy. Psychological Medicine, 32, 763-782.

Seckinger, R. A., & Amador, X. F. (2001). Cognitive-behavioral therapy in schizophrenia. Journal of Psychiatric Practice, 7, 173-184.

Chapter 12: Personality Disorders

LEARNING OBJECTIVES

After reading and studying this chapter, you should be able to:

1. Identify the differences between personality disorders and acute disorders.

2. Identify the three clusters of personality disorders, the disorders in each cluster, and the ways in which the disorders in each cluster are related.

3. Discuss the criticisms of the DSM's approach to classifying personality disorders.

4. Discuss the controversies that surround the personality disorders, including claims that gender and ethnic/racial bias impact them.

5. Identify the similarities and differences between schizophrenia and the odd-eccentric personality disorders.

6. Describe the key symptoms and characteristics of each personality disorder, the theories that attempt to explain it, and the approaches used to treat it.

7. Discuss why some of the personality disorders (such as antisocial personality disorder) are especially difficult to treat.

8. Identify the differences between avoidant personality disorder, social phobia, and schizoid personality disorder.

9. Identify the similarities and differences between obsessive-compulsive disorder and obsessive-compulsive personality disorder.

10. Describe alternative conceptualizations of the personality disorders.

ESSENTIAL IDEAS

I. Defining and diagnosing personality disorders

    A. A personality disorder is a long-standing pattern of behaviors, thoughts, and feelings that is highly maladaptive for the individual or for people around him or her.

    B. A personality disorder must be present continuously from adolescence or early adulthood into adulthood.

    C. Personality disorders are listed on Axis II of the DSM-IV-TR.

D. The DSM-IV-TR divides the personality disorders into three clusters: the odd-eccentric disorders, the dramatic-emotional disorders, and the anxious-fearful disorders.

E. Some theorists object to the DSM's classification of personality disorders because: (1) it treats these disorders as categories; (2) the diagnostic criteria for these disorders overlap to a large extent; and (3) the diagnostic criteria have low reliability.

F. The DSM-IV-TR construction of personality disorders may be gender biased because some criteria appear to represent extreme stereotypes of masculine or feminine behavior. These criteria may also fail to consider how men and women can exhibit symptoms in different ways.

II. Odd-eccentric personality disorders

A. People diagnosed with the odd-eccentric personality disorders—paranoid, schizoid, and schizotypal personality disorders—have odd thought processes, emotional reactions, and behaviors similar to those of people with schizophrenia, but they retain their grasp on reality.

B. People diagnosed with paranoid personality disorder are chronically suspicious of others but maintain their grasp on reality.

C. People diagnosed with schizoid personality disorder are emotionally cold and distant from others and have great trouble forming interpersonal relationships.

D. People diagnosed with schizotypal personality disorders have a variety of odd beliefs and perceptual experiences but also maintain their grasp on reality.

E. These personality disorders, especially schizotypal personality disorder, have been linked to familial histories of schizophrenia and some of the biological abnormalities of schizophrenia.

F. People diagnosed with these disorders tend not to seek treatment, but when they do, therapists pay close attention to the therapeutic relationship and help the clients learn to reality-test their unusual thinking.

G. Antipsychotics may help people with schizotypal personality disorder reduce their odd thinking.

III. Dramatic-emotional personality disorders

A. People with dramatic-emotional personality disorders—antisocial, borderline, histrionic, and narcissistic personality disorders—have histories of unstable relationships and emotional experiences and of dramatic, erratic behavior.

B. People with antisocial personality disorder regularly violate the basic rights of others, and many engage in criminal acts.

C. Antisocial personality disorder may have strong biological roots but is also associated with harsh and non-supportive parenting.

D. People with borderline personality disorder vacillate between all good and all bad evaluations of themselves and others.

E. People with histrionic and narcissistic personality disorders act in a flamboyant manner. People with histrionic personality disorder are overly dependent and solicitious of others, whereas people with narcissistic personality disorder are dismissive of others.

F. None of these personality disorders responds consistently well to current treatments.

IV. Anxious-fearful personality disorders

A. People with the anxious-fearful personality disorders—avoidant, dependent, and obsessive-compulsive personality disorders—are chronically fearful or concerned.

B. People with avoidant personality disorder worry about being criticized.

C. People with dependent personality disorder worry about being abandoned.

D. People with obsessive-compulsive personality disorder are locked into rigid routines of behavior and become anxious when their routines are violated.

E. Some children may be born with temperamental predispositions toward shy and avoidant behaviors, or childhood anxiety may contribute to dependent personalities.

F. These disorders may also arise from a lack of nurturing parenting and basic fears about one's ability to function competently.

V. Alternative conceptualizations of personality disorders

A. Some critics of the categorical models of personality disorders in the DSM-IV-TR have suggested that the personality disorders represent extremes of normal personality traits. These critics argue for dimensional, rather than categorical, models of these disorders.

B. One scheme for organizing the personality disorders along dimensions takes off from the Big 5 personality traits: neuroticism, extraversion, openness to experience, agreeableness, and conscientiousness.

KEY TERMS AND GUIDED REVIEW

Defining and Diagnosing Personality Disorders

<u>Key Terms</u>

personality:

personality disorder:

<u>Guided Review</u>

1. Describe some ways in which personality disorders differ from Axis I disorders.

2. Describe the three clusters of personality disorders.

3. What are some of the criticisms of the DSM conceptualization of personality disorders?

4. Describe some of the problems associated with gender and ethnic/racial bias in the diagnosis of personality disorders. What solutions have theorists proposed to manage these problems?

Odd-Eccentric Personality Disorders

<u>Key Terms</u>

odd-eccentric personality disorders:

paranoid personality disorder:

schizoid personality disorder:

schizotypal personality disorder:

<u>Guided Review</u>

1. What are some characteristics of people with paranoid personality disorder?

2. How does cognitive theory attempt to explain paranoid personality disorder?

3. Describe some techniques used to treat paranoid personality disorder.

4. What are some characteristics of people with schizoid personality disorder?

5. What are some techniques used to treat schizoid personality disorder?

6. Describe the oddities in cognition found in people with schizotypal personality disorder.

7. What are some biological abnormalities found in people with schizotypal personality disorder?

8. What are some techniques used to treat schizotypal personality disorder?

Dramatic-Emotional Personality Disorders

Key Terms

dramatic-emotional personality disorders:

antisocial personality disorder:

psychopathy:

serotonin:

executive functions:

borderline personality disorder:

splitting:

dialectical behavior therapy:

histrionic personality disorder:

narcissistic personality disorder:

Guided Review

1. What are some characteristics of people with antisocial personality disorder?

2. How does antisocial personality disorder differ from psychopathy?

2. What is the evidence that genetics influence antisocial behavior?

3. Describe some of the biological and cognitive deficits associated with antisocial behavior.

4. Why are people with antisocial personality disorder difficult to treat, and what are some techniques used in the treatment of this disorder?

5. What are some characteristics of people with borderline personality disorder?

6. What other conditions tend to be associated with borderline personality disorder?

7. Describe the object relations theory of borderline personality disorder.

8. What is Linehan's theory of borderline personality disorder?

9. Describe some techniques used to treat borderline personality disorder.

10. What are some characteristics of people with histrionic personality disorder?

11. What are some techniques used to treat histrionic personality disorder?

12. What are some characteristics of people with narcissistic personality disorder?

13. Summarize the theories of narcissistic personality disorder.

14. Why do people with narcissistic personality disorder rarely seek treatment, and what techniques are used to treat this disorder?

Anxious-Fearful Personality Disorders

Key Terms

anxious-fearful personality disorders:

avoidant personality disorder:

dependent personality disorder:

obsessive-compulsive personality disorder:

Guided Review

1. What are some characteristics of people with avoidant personality disorder?

2. Describe some theories of avoidant personality disorder.

3. What are some techniques used in the treatment of avoidant personality disorder?

4. What are some characteristics of people with dependent personality disorder?

5. Describe some techniques used in the treatment of dependent personality disorder.

6. What are some characteristics of people with obsessive-compulsive personality disorder?

7. Describe some theories of obsessive-compulsive personality disorder.

8. What are some techniques used in the treatment of obsessive-compulsive personality disorder?

Alternative Conceptualizations of Personality Disorders

<u>Key Terms</u>

five-factor model:

<u>Guided Review</u>

1. What is the five-factor model and how might it improve the classification of personality disorders?

2. What are some strengths and weaknesses of dimensional models?

CASE EXAMPLE
Read the following description and answer the questions below:

Horace had lost his job at the post office because he often did not show up for work and when he was at work, he was often unable to complete the tasks he was assigned. He was distressed over his job loss and sought help at a community mental health center.

At the initial interview, Horace was distant and somewhat distrustful of the interviewer. He mentioned that he had few friends. He also did not have a good relationship with his family, and spent long hours thinking angry thoughts about his brother, but then worrying that these thoughts would somehow actually cause harm to his brother.

Horace had a lot on his mind. He told the interviewer he had spent an hour and a half at the pet store debating which dog food to buy, and described in great, irrelevant detail the relative merits of the different brands. He also said he had spent two days studying the washing instructions on a new pair of pants. He wondered whether "wash before wearing" meant that the jeans were to be washed before wearing the first time, or did they need to be washed each time before they were worn. He felt that this question was of great importance, both to him and to the interviewer. Horace also described how he often bought several different brands of the same item, such as different kinds of can openers, and then would keep them in their original bags in his closet, expecting that at some future time he would find them useful. He was usually reluctant to spend money on things that he actually needed, however, even though he had plenty of money. He could recite from memory his most recent monthly bank statement, including the amount of every check and the running balance as each check was written. He knew his balance on any particular day, but sometimes got anxious if he considered whether a certain check or deposit had actually cleared.

He asked the interviewer whether he might be asked to participate in groups if he were to receive counseling. He said that groups made him nervous. He was afraid that he might reveal too much information about himself, which group members would then use to take advantage of him. (Adapted from Spitzer, Gibbon, Skodol, Williams, and First, 1994, pp. 289-290).

1. This person has symptoms that suggest three possible personality disorder diagnoses. What are these symptoms and what are the three possible diagnoses?

2. Which of these three diagnoses do you think best fits this person, and why?

3. Some of this person's thought patterns sound like obsessions. Are they obsessions? Why or why not?

CHAPTER TEST

A. <u>Multiple Choice</u>. Choose the **best answer** to each question below.

1. Personality disorders

    A. must be present continuously since childhood.
    B. are often difficult to diagnose reliably.
    C. are listed on Axis III.
    D. are more likely to cause people to seek treatment than are acute disorders.

2. Women are more likely than men to be diagnosed with all of the following <u>except</u>:

    A. histrionic personality disorder.
    B. borderline personality disorder.
    C. dependent personality disorder.
    D. avoidant personality disorder.

3. All of the following are odd-eccentric personality disorders <u>except</u>:

    A. avoidant personality disorder.
    B. schizotypal personality disorder.
    C. schizoid personality disorder.
    D. paranoid personality disorder.

4. It is recommended that to treat _____ personality disorder, a therapist should be extremely straightforward and not attempt to develop a warm, close relationship with the client.

    A. schizoid
    B. narcissistic
    C. paranoid
    D. avoidant

5. People with _____ personality disorder lack any desire to form interpersonal relationships and are emotionally cold in interactions with others. They view relationships with others as unrewarding, messy, and intrusive.

    A. obsessive-compulsive
    B. avoidant
    C. schizoid
    D. schizotypal

6. All of the following are cognitive oddities in people with schizotypal personality disorder except:

    A. ideas of reference.
    B. hallucinations.
    C. tangential, circumstantial, or vague speech.
    D. magical thinking.

7. All of the following are abnormalities found in both schizophrenia and schizotypal personality disorder except:

    A. deficits in sustained attention.
    B. abnormally high levels of dopamine.
    C. enlarged ventricles.
    D. decreased activity in the temporal lobe.

8. All of the following are dramatic-emotional personality disorders except:

    A. borderline personality disorder.
    B. antisocial personality disorder.
    C. dependent personality disorder.
    D. narcissistic personality disorder.

9. People with antisocial personality disorder exhibit all of the following except:

    A. deficits in the parietal lobes of the brain.
    B. poor impulse control.
    C. deficits in executive functions.
    D. difficulty inhibiting impulsive behaviors.

10. Most people with antisocial personality disorder:

    A. are women.
    B. abuse substances.
    C. attempt suicide.
    D. are remorseful about their criminal behavior.

11. People with _____ personality disorder tend to see themselves and other people as either "all good" or "all bad"—a process known as splitting.

      A. antisocial
      B. borderline
      C. paranoid
      D. narcissistic

12. People with _____ are heavy users of mental health services, in contrast to people with other personality disorders.

      A. borderline
      B. antisocial
      C. avoidant
      D. narcissistic

13. Both _____ and _____ personality disorders are correlated with low levels of serotonin.

      A. avoidant; dependent
      B. paranoid; antisocial
      C. antisocial; borderline
      D. obsessive-compulsive; avoidant

14. The development of _____ personality disorder is believed to stem from overindulgence and overvaluation by significant others during childhood.

      A. dependent
      B. histrionic
      C. borderline
      D. narcissistic

15. Dialectical behavior therapy is used in the treatment of

      A. obsessive-compulsive personality disorder.
      B. schizotypal personality disorder.
      C. antisocial personality disorder.
      D. borderline personality disorder.

16. Avoidant personality disorder shares many characteristics with

      A. social phobia.
      B. generalized anxiety disorder.
      C. histrionic personality disorder.
      D. cyclothymic disorder.

17. Treatment for _____ personality disorder might include mastery of a hierarchy of increasingly difficult independent actions that clients gradually attempt on their own.

  A. obsessive-compulsive
  B. dependent
  C. avoidant
  D. paranoid

18. Men are more likely than women to be diagnosed with all of the following except:

  A. paranoid personality disorder.
  B. antisocial personality disorder.
  C. histrionic personality disorder.
  D. obsessive-compulsive personality disorder.

19. Individuals with which personality disorder would be most likely to say, "Mistakes are not acceptable"?

  A. Antisocial personality disorder
  B. Paranoid personality disorder
  C. Obsessive-compulsive personality disorder
  D. Dependent personality disorder

20. Individuals low on _____ are cynical, rude, suspicious, uncooperative, and irritable.

  A. conscientiousness
  B. openness to experience
  C. extraversion
  D. agreeableness

B. True-False. Select T (True) or F (False) below.

1. When clinicians use structured interviews rather than unstructured interviews, they tend to find that women are more often diagnosed with histrionic, borderline, and dependent personality disorders, whereas men are more often diagnosed with antisocial personality disorder.
    T   F

2. African Americans are more likely than Caucasians to be diagnosed with schizotypal personality disorder.   T   F

3. There is strong, consistent evidence that testosterone plays a role in antisocial behavior.
    T   F

4. Research has found a genetic link between avoidant personality disorder and schizophrenia.
    T   F

5. The relatives of people with borderline personality disorder have high rates of mood disorders.

    T   F

C. <u>Short Answer Questions</u>.

1. What are some of the criticisms of the DSM approach to classifying personality disorders? Give an example of an alternative classification system.

2. Describe Linehan's dialectical behavior therapy for borderline personality disorder.

3. Which personality disorders appear to be related to schizophrenia? Explain the ways in which these disorders are similar to and different from schizophrenia.

4. Why do some theorists believe that the DSM personality disorder criteria are gender-biased? What are some ways in which this bias might be reduced?

5. Give examples of how some of the personality disorders described in the chapter may be somewhat adaptive in certain cultures.

ANSWER KEY

Case Example
1. Schizotypal personality disorder: odd beliefs and magical thinking, over-elaborate speaking, paranoia, lack of close friends, social anxiety; schizoid personality disorder: absence of close friends; obsessive-compulsive personality disorder: obsessional thoughts and compulsive behaviors about purchases.
2. Meets all criteria for schizotypal personality disorder, but not for other two.
3. Probably not obsessions because they are ego-syntonic.

Multiple Choice
1. B
2. D
3. A
4. C
5. C
6. B
7. D
8. C
9. A
10. B
11. B
12. A
13. C
14. A
15. D
16. A
17. B
18. C
19. C
20. D

True-False
1. T
2. T
3. F
4. F
5. T

Short Answer Questions
1. See pp. 424–425, 452–454.
2. See pp. 443–444.
3. See pp. 428–434.
4. See pp. 426–428.
5. See p. 436.

Additional Readings on Chapter 12 Topics

Davis, R. D. (1999). Millon: Essentials of his science, theory, classification, assessment, and theory. <u>Journal of Personality Assessment, 72,</u> 330-352.

Koerner, K., & Linehan, M. M. (2000). Research on dialectical behavior therapy for patients with borderline personality disorder. <u>Psychiatric Clinics of North American, 23,</u> 151-167.

Ryder, A. G., & Bagby, R. M. (1999). Diagnostic viability of depressive personality disorder: Theoretical and conceptual issues. <u>Journal of Personality Disorders, 13,</u> 99-117.

* Note that depressive personality disorder is not included among the personality disorders in DSM-IV-TR, but is listed instead under "Criteria sets and axes provided for further study."

Chapter 13: Childhood Disorders

LEARNING OBJECTIVES

After reading and studying this chapter, you should be able to:

1. Identify the symptoms of attention-deficit/hyperactivity disorder (ADHD), describe how it affects a child's social and intellectual functioning, and discuss how it affects children as they enter adolescence and adulthood.

2. Discuss the genetic and neurological contributors to ADHD, and the other psychopathological conditions associated with ADHD.

3. Describe the drug therapies and psychosocial therapies for ADHD.

4. Discuss the similarities and differences between conduct disorder, oppositional defiant disorder, and ADHD.

5. Discuss the symptoms and course of conduct disorder and oppositional defiant disorder.

6. Describe the biological and psychosocial contributors to conduct disorder and oppositional defiant disorder.

7. Describe the drug therapies and psychotherapies used to treat conduct and oppositional defiant disorder.

8. Identify the symptoms of separation anxiety disorder, and describe adult outcomes for children with this disorder.

9. Discuss the genetic factors and parenting practices that may lead to separation anxiety disorder.

10. Discuss ways to treat separation anxiety disorder.

11. Identify the diagnostic criteria for enuresis and encopresis, the theories that explain their development, and the most effective treatments for these disorders.

12. Distinguish among learning disorders, motor skills disorders, and communication disorders.

13. Discuss what is required for a diagnosis of mental retardation, the difference between organic and cultural-familial mental retardation, and how the symptoms of the disorder vary in severity from mild to moderate to severe to profound.

14. Discuss and distinguish among the numerous diseases, maternal behaviors, and aspects of pregnancy and birth that can lead to mental retardation.

15. Discuss the social factors that may contribute to mental retardation.

16. Discuss some of the effective interventions for mental retardation.

17. Describe the deficits exhibited by autistic children.

18. Distinguish among autism, Rett's disorder, childhood disintegrative disorder, and Asperger's disorder.

19. Discuss the genetic and biological causes of autism.

20. Discuss the drugs used to treat the symptoms of autism, and the behavioral methods used to treat autistic children.

ESSENTIAL IDEAS

I. Behavior disorders

A. The behavior disorders include attention-deficit/hyperactivity disorder, conduct disorder, and oppositional defiant disorder.

B. Children with attention-deficit/hyperactivity disorder are inattentive, impulsive, and overactive. They often do not do well in school, and their relationships with their peers are extremely impaired.

C. Some children with attention-deficit/hyperactivity disorder grow out of this disorder, but some continue to show the symptoms into adulthood, and they are at high risk for conduct problems and emotional problems throughout their lives.

D. The two therapies that are effective in treating ADHD are stimulant drugs and behavior therapies that teach children how to control their behaviors. The combination of medications and behavior therapies appears to lead to the most long-lasting improvement.

E. Children with conduct disorder engage in behaviors that severely violate societal norms, including chronic lying, stealing, and violence toward others.

F. Children with oppositional defiant disorder engage in antisocial behaviors that are less severe than those of conduct disorder but indicate a negative, irritable approach to others.

G. Some children outgrow oppositional defiant disorder, but a subset develops full conduct disorder.

H. Children who develop conduct disorder often continue to engage in antisocial behaviors into adulthood and have high rates of criminal activity and drug abuse.

I. Neurological deficits may be involved in conduct disorder. These deficits may make it more difficult for children with this disorder to learn from reinforcements and punishments and to control their behaviors.

J. Children with conduct disorder tend to have parents who are neglectful much of the time and become violent when annoyed with them.

K. Children with conduct disorder tend to think about interactions with others in ways that contribute to their aggressive reactions.

L. Drug therapies are sometimes used to help children with conduct disorder control their behavior, and cognitive-behavioral therapies help them learn to interpret and respond to situations differently.

II. Separation anxiety disorder

A. Children can suffer from all the emotional disorders, including depression and all the anxiety disorders. Separation anxiety disorder is one disorder specific to children.

B. Children with separation anxiety disorder are excessively fearful about separation from primary caregivers. They may become extremely agitated or ill when they anticipate separation, and they may curtail usual activities to avoid separation.

C. Separation anxiety disorder appears to be associated with a family history of anxiety disorders.

D. Children who are behaviorally inhibited as infants appear at risk for separation anxiety disorder as adults.

E. Parents may enhance a vulnerability to separation anxiety disorder by their reactions to children's distress.

F. Cognitive-behavioral therapies can help children with separation anxiety disorder quiet their anxieties and resume everyday activities.

III. Elimination disorders

A. Enuresis is persistent uncontrolled wetting by children who have attained bladder control.

B. Enuresis runs in families and has been attributed to a variety of biological causes. Psychodynamic theories attribute it to emotional distress. Behavioral theories attribute it to poor toilet training.

C. Antidepressants help to reduce enuresis in the short term, but not in the long term, and carry significant side effects.

D. Behavioral methods that help the child learn to awaken and go to the bathroom can help to reduce nighttime enuresis.

E. Encopresis is persistent uncontrolled soiling by children who have attained control of defecation.

F. Encopresis typically begins after one or more episodes of constipation, which create distention in the colon and decrease a child's ability to detect needed bowel movements.

G. Medical management and behavioral techniques can help reduce encopresis.

IV. Disorders of cognitive, motor, and communication skills

A. Learning disorders include reading disorder (inability to read, also known as dyslexia), mathematics disorder (inability to learn math), and disorder of written expression (inability to write).

B. Developmental coordination disorder involves deficits in fundamental motor skills.

C. Communication disorders include expressive language disorder (an inability to express oneself through language), mixed receptive-expressive language disorder (an inability to express oneself through language or to understand the language of others), phonological disorder (the use of speech sounds inappropriate for the age and dialect), and stuttering (deficits in word fluency).

D. Some of these disorders, particularly reading disorder and stuttering, may have genetic roots. Many other factors have been implicated in these disorders, but they are not well understood.

E. Treatment usually focuses on building skills in problem areas through specialized training and computerized exercises.

V. Mental retardation

A. Mental retardation is defined as subaverage intellectual functioning, indexed by an IQ score of under 70 and deficits in adaptive behavioral functioning. There are four levels of mental retardation, ranging from mild to profound.

B. A number of biological factors are implicated in mental retardation, including metabolic disorders (PKU, Tay-Sachs disease); chromosomal disorders (Down syndrome, Fragile X, Trisomy 13, and Trisomy 18); prenatal exposure to rubella, herpes, syphilis, or drugs (especially alcohol); premature delivery; and head traumas (such as those arising from being violently shaken).

C. There is some evidence that intensive and comprehensive educational interventions, administered very early in life, can help to decrease the level of mental retardation.

D. Controversy exists over whether children with mental retardation should be put in special education classes or mainstreamed into normal classrooms.

VI. Pervasive developmental disorders

A. The pervasive developmental disorders are characterized by severe and lasting impairment in several areas of development, including social interaction, communication, everyday behaviors, interests, and activities. They include Asperger's disorder, Rett's disorder, childhood disintegrative disorder, and autism.

B. Autism is characterized by significant interpersonal, communication, and behavioral deficits. Two-thirds of autistic children score in the mentally retarded range on IQ tests.

C. There is wide variation in the outcome of autism, although the majority of autistic children must have continual care as adults. The best predictors of a good outcome in autism are an IQ above 50 and language development before the age of 6.

D. Biological causes of autism may include a genetic predisposition to cognitive impairment, central nervous system damage, prenatal complications, and neurotransmitter imbalances.

E. Drugs reduce some behaviors in autism but do not eliminate the core of the disorder.

F. Behavior therapy is used to reduce inappropriate and self-injurious behaviors and to encourage prosocial behaviors in children with autism.

KEY TERMS AND GUIDED REVIEW

Guided Review

1. Describe the relationship between stress and the development of psychological disorders in children.

2. Describe some ways in which temperament is related to psychological disorders in children.

Behavior Disorders

Key Terms

attention deficit/hyperactivity disorder (ADHD):

conduct disorder:

oppositional defiant disorder:

1. Describe the three subtypes of ADHD.

2. What are some problems that children with ADHD tend to have in addition to the ADHD itself?

3. How common is ADHD, and how do the rates of ADHD vary by gender?

4. Does ADHD persist into adulthood? What are some problems experienced by adults who had ADHD as children?

5. What brain areas and neurotransmitters are involved in ADHD?

6. What conditions tend to run in the families of children who develop ADHD?

7. What pregnancy-related and familial factors are associated with ADHD?

8. Describe the effective treatments for ADHD.

9. Describe the symptoms of conduct disorder.

10. What are some problems experienced by adults who had conduct disorder as children?

11. How does oppositional defiant disorder differ from conduct disorder?

12. How do the rates and presentation of conduct disorder differ by gender?

13. What are some biological contributors to conduct and oppositional defiant disorder?

14. Describe some sociocultural contributors to conduct and oppositional defiant disorder.

15. Describe how children with conduct disorder tend to process information about social interactions.

16. What drug and psychological therapies appear to be effective for children with conduct disorder? How does race/ethnicity appear to impact treatment decisions for children with conduct disorder?

Separation Anxiety Disorder

Key Terms

separation anxiety disorder:

Guided Review

1. Describe how children with separation anxiety disorder differ from normal children.

2. Describe some long-term effects of separation anxiety disorder.

3. What is behavioral inhibition, and how does it relate to separation anxiety disorder?

4. What are some psychological and sociocultural contributors to separation anxiety disorder?

5. Describe how separation anxiety may be effectively treated.

Elimination Disorders

Key Terms

elimination disorders:

enuresis:

encopresis:

Guided Review

1. What is enuresis? How common is it?

2. What are some biological, psychodynamic, and behavioral contributors to enuresis?

3. What treatments are available for enuresis?

4. What is encopresis? How common is it?

5. Describe how encopresis may be effectively treated.

Disorders of Cognitive, Motor, and Communication Skills

Key Terms

learning disorders:

reading disorder:

mathematics disorder:

disorder of written expression:

motor skills disorder:

developmental coordination disorder:

communication disorders:

expressive language disorder:

mixed receptive-expressive language disorder:

phonological disorder:

stuttering:

<u>Guided Review</u>

1. How do learning disorders impact children and adults?

2. What are the symptoms of developmental coordination disorder?

3. How are expressive language disorder, mixed receptive-expressive language disorder, phonological disorder, and stuttering similar to and different from one another?

Mental Retardation

<u>Key Terms</u>

mental retardation:

phenylketonuria (PKU):

Tay-Sachs disease:

Down syndrome:

Fragile X syndrome:

Trisomy 13:

Trisomy 18:

fetal alcohol syndrome:

shaken baby syndrome:

<u>Guided Review</u>

1. What besides a low IQ must be present for someone to be diagnosed with mental retardation?

2. What are the differences among mild, moderate, severe, and profound mental retardation?

3. Describe some of the genetic conditions that can cause mental retardation.

4. Describe some of the prenatal contributors to mental retardation.

5. What are the consequences of shaking a baby?

6. What are some sociocultural contributors to mental retardation?

7. What behavioral and drug therapies appear to be helpful for mentally retarded children?

8. Describe the Infant Health and Development Program. Was it effective, and if so, why?

9. What are some alternatives to drug or behavior therapy for mentally retarded people?

Pervasive Developmental Disorders

<u>Key Terms</u>

pervasive developmental disorders:

autism:

Asperger's disorder:

Rett's disorder:

childhood disintegrative disorder:

echolalia:

<u>Guided Review</u>

1. What are the symptoms of autism?

2. Describe the course of autism and the factors associated with better outcomes.

3. How does Asperger's disorder differ from autism?

4. Describe how theory of mind relates to autism.

5. What are some biological contributors to autism?

6. Describe some of the treatments that are helpful for children with autism.

CASE EXAMPLE
Read the following description and answer the questions below:

Karen is a difficult child. At school, she rarely listens to her teacher and often gets up from her chair and wanders around the classroom. When her teacher reprimands her for this, Karen either blatantly ignores the teacher, or says something "smart" to the teacher, such as, "I'm too bored to sit in my seat." Even when she sits in her seat, Karen often disrupts the other children, talking loudly at them when they are trying to concentrate, sometimes insulting them. Karen doesn't finish her school assignments most of the time. After just a few minutes of working on an assignment, Karen declares that it is "stupid" and gets out of her seat to find something more interesting to do. On the playground, few children want to play with Karen because she throws temper tantrums if she doesn't get to do things exactly her way.

At home, Karen frequently disobeys her parents, even though she is punished harshly when she is caught disobeying. Karen is prone to dangerous activities—one night she crawled out her bedroom window onto the roof of her house, "just because I wanted to." If siblings annoy her, Karen is prone to hitting them, even the brother who is much older and bigger than her. This brother tends to taunt Karen, calling her dumb because she doesn't do well in school. When Karen strikes this brother, he hits her back. He has given her a black eye twice.

1. What two diagnoses may fit Karen's symptoms? Can Karen be given both of these diagnoses?

2. List the symptoms of each of these disorders that Karen shows.

3. What family factors may contribute to Karen's behavior?

CHAPTER TEST

A. <u>Multiple Choice</u>. Choose the **best answer** to each question below.

1. All of the following are classified as pervasive developmental disorders <u>except</u>:

    A. autism.
    B. Asperger's disorder.
    C. selective mutism.
    D. childhood disintegrative disorder.

2. The symptoms of ADHD fall into all of the following categories <u>except</u>:

A. inattention.
B. defiance.
C. impulsivity.
D. hyperactivity.

3. Boys are more likely than girls to develop all of the following <u>except</u>:

A. separation anxiety disorder.
B. encopresis.
C. ADHD.
D. autism.

4. Which of the following brain areas has been implicated in ADHD?

A. The occipital lobes
B. The thalamus
C. The frontal lobes
D. The hippocampus

5. Which of the following has <u>not</u> been found to predispose children to ADHD?

A. Premature delivery
B. Consumption of large amounts of sugar
C. Maternal nicotine consumption
D. Exposure to high concentrations of lead

6. Which of the following statements about differences between conduct and oppositional defiant disorder is <u>false</u>?

A. Conduct disorder is more severe than oppositional defiant disorder.
B. Boys are three times more likely than girls to develop conduct disorder, but the rates of oppositional defiant disorder do not differ by gender.
C. Twin studies suggest that both conduct and oppositional defiant disorder are influenced by genetics.
D. Oppositional defiant disorder is diagnosed at an earlier age than conduct disorder.

7. All of the following are associated with conduct disorder <u>except</u>:

A. lower levels of cortisol.
B. ADHD.
C. maternal exposure to toxins during pregnancy.
D. living in a rural area.

8. Henry has been having problems in school lately. When his gym teacher told him to do 20 push-ups because he called another child a "sissy," Henry blew up and argued with his gym teacher. His teachers say that at times, Henry refuses to pay attention to them. At home, Henry

often steals his sister's toys and hides them just to annoy her. He is very jealous of his sister, and pouts whenever she does well at something, calling her "the favorite child." Henry's problems are most consistent with a diagnosis of

    A. ADHD.
    B. oppositional defiant disorder.
    C. conduct disorder.
    D. separation anxiety disorder.

9. All of the following are symptoms of separation anxiety disorder except:

    A. persistent and excessive worry about losing, or harm coming to, caregivers.
    B. excessively fearful about being alone.
    C. repeated nightmares involving themes of separation.
    D. excessive sleeping when caregivers are not present.

10. Which of the following is not associated with separation anxiety disorder?

    A. Decreased levels of dopamine
    B. Behavioral inhibition
    C. Having a family that is close-knit and does not encourage independence
    D. Exposure to traumatic events

11. Encopresis

    A. must occur at least twice a week for 3 months to be diagnosed.
    B. may be effectively treated with the bell and pad method.
    C. is less common than enuresis.
    D. tends to run in families.

12. Dyslexia is a term often used to refer to

    A. reading disorder.
    B. receptive language disorder.
    C. phonological disorder.
    D. disorder of reading comprehension.

13. Which of the following disorders is least common?

    A. Reading disorder
    B. Developmental coordination disorder
    C. Expressive language disorder
    D. Mathematics disorder

14. Children with _____ mental retardation have very limited vocabularies, speak in two-to-three-word sentences, and have IQ scores between 20 and 35.

A. mild
B. moderate
C. severe
D. profound

15. Which of the following childhood diseases resembles Alzheimer's disease in that both consist of tangles and plaques on neurons in the brain as well as memory loss and an inability to care for oneself?

A. Down syndrome
B. Fragile X syndrome
C. Phenylketonuria
D. Fetal alcohol syndrome

16. A disorder marked by deficits in social interactions and in activities and interests, but not in language or basic cognitive skills, is known as

A. autism.
B. Rett's disorder.
C. Asperger's disorder.
D. childhood disintegrative disorder.

17. Children with _____ typically have deficits in theory of mind and symbolic play.

A. conduct disorder
B. autism
C. ADHD
D. oppositional defiant disorder

18. Which of the following childhood diseases is the most common cause of mental retardation?

A. Down Syndrome
B. Fragile X syndrome
C. Trisomy 18
D. Phenylketonuria

19. All of the following are groups of deficits in autism except:

A. activities and interests.
B. communication.
C. social interactions.
D. inattention.

20. The best predictors of outcome in autism are

A. the child's IQ and language development before age 6.
B. the child's emotional development before age 6.
C. the child's capacity for nonverbal communication.
D. the quality of parenting the child receives.

B. <u>True-False</u>. Select T (True) or F (False) below.

1. Most children with ADHD have a history of brain injury. T   F

2. African American and European American children have similar rates of conduct disorder.
    T   F

3. When a child obtains an IQ score less than 70, he or she meets criteria for mental retardation.
    T   F

4. Stimulants seem to be effective for the treatment of ADHD because they increase levels of GABA in the brain.   T   F

5. The majority of children with autism go on to develop schizophrenia as adults.   T   F

C. <u>Short Answer Questions</u>.

1. Describe how cognitive-behavioral techniques may be used to treat conduct disorder.

2. What are some ways in which ADHD and conduct disorder are related?

3. Describe some of the methods used to treat mental retardation.

4. Compare and contrast enuresis and encopresis in terms of their symptoms, prevalence, and effective treatments.

5. Compare drug treatments and behavior treatments for ADHD, and describe the treatments believed to result in the best outcomes for children with ADHD.

ANSWER KEY

<u>Case Example</u>
1. Attention deficit disorder and oppositional defiant disorder. Yes, Karen can be given both of these diagnoses.
2. ADHD: not listening to the teacher, getting up and walking around class, difficulty being quiet in class, disrupting the other children, temper tantrums, dangerous impulsive behaviors like going out on the roof and striking a larger brother. Oppositional defiant disorder: chronically defies teacher and parents, deliberately annoys other children and siblings, easily annoyed, often loses temper, argues with adults.
3. Use of harsh punishment by parents, modeling of aggressive behaviors by brother.

<u>Multiple Choice</u>
1. C
2. B
3. A
4. C
5. B
6. B
7. D
8. B
9. D
10. A
11. C
12. A
13. D
14. C
15. A
16. C
17. B
18. A
19. D
20. A

<u>True-False</u>
1. F
2. T
3. F (Importantly, this is not the only criterion for mental retardation)
4. F
5. F

<u>Short Answer Questions</u>
1. See p. 477.
2. See pp. 464–478.

3. See pp. 493–496.
4. See pp. 483–485.
5. See pp. 469–470.

Additional Readings on Chapter 13 Topics

Barkley, R. A., et al. (2002). Consensus statement on ADHD. European Child and Adolescent Psychiatry, 11, 96-98.

Lovaas, O. I., & Smith, T. (1989). A comprehensive behavioral theory of autistic children: Paradigm for research and treatment. Journal of Behavior Therapy and Experimental Psychiatry, 20, 17-29.

Moffitt, T. E., Caspi, A., Harrington, H., & Milne, B. J. (2002). Males on the life-course-persistent and adolescence-limited antisocial pathways: Follow-up at age 26 years. Development and Psychopathology, 14, 179-207.

Chapter 14: Cognitive Disorders and Life-Span Issues

LEARNING OBJECTIVES
After reading and studying this chapter, you should be able to:

1. Explain why the cognitive disorders are no longer known as "organic brain disorders."

2. Identify when a set of symptoms should be diagnosed as a cognitive disorder, and when it should not be.

3. Identify the types of cognitive impairment in dementia.

4. Describe the symptoms of Alzheimer's disease.

5. Identify and describe the brain changes that occur in Alzheimer's disease and the conditions thought to cause them.

6. Discuss the evidence for a genetic contribution to Alzheimer's disease.

7. Describe vascular dementia and identify its causes.

8. Describe the potential causes of traumatic brain injuries.

9. Describe the symptoms of Parkinson's disease, HIV-associated dementia, and Huntington's disease.

10. Discuss the available treatments for dementia.

11. Discuss how culture and gender may affect dementia.

12. Identify the symptoms of delirium, their typical progression, and the conditions that make a diagnosis likely.

13. Discuss the ways in which delirium can be treated.

14. Distinguish between anterograde and retrograde amnesia.

15. Identify how amnesic disorders may be treated.

16. Discuss older adults' experiences of anxiety disorders, depression, and substance use disorders.

ESSENTIAL IDEAS

I. Dementia

A. Dementia is typically a permanent deterioration in cognitive functioning, often accompanied by emotional changes.

B. The five types of cognitive impairments in dementia are memory impairment, aphasia, apraxia, agnosia, and loss of executive functioning.

C. The most common type of dementia is due to Alzheimer's disease.

D. The brains of Alzheimer's patients show neurofibrillary tangles, plaques made up of amyloid protein, and cortical atrophy.

E. Recent theories of Alzheimer's disease focus on three genes that might contribute to the buildup of amyloid in the brains of Alzheimer's disease patients.

F. Dementia can also be caused by cerebrovascular disorder, head injury, and progressive disorders such as Parkinson's disease, HIV disease, Huntington's disease, and more rarely, Pick's disease, Creutzfeldt-Jakob disease, and a number of other medical conditions. Finally, chronic drug abuse and the nutritional deficiencies that often accompany it can lead to dementia.

G. Some drugs help to reduce the cognitive symptoms and accompanying depression, anxiety, and psychotic symptoms in some patients with dementia.

H. Gender, culture, and education all play roles in vulnerability to dementia.

II. Delirium

A. Delirium is characterized by disorientation, recent memory loss, and clouding of consciousness.

B. The onset of delirium can be either sudden or slow.

C. The many causes of delirium include medical diseases, the trauma of surgery, illicit drugs, medications, high fever, and infections.

D. Delirium must be addressed immediately by treating its underlying causes, to prevent brain damage and to prevent people from hurting themselves.

III. Amnesia

A. The amnesic disorders are characterized only by memory loss.

B. Retrograde amnesia is loss of memory for past events. Anterograde amnesia is the inability to remember new information.

C. Amnesia can be caused by brain damage due to strokes, head injuries, chronic nutritional deficiencies, exposure to toxins (such as through carbon monoxide poisoning), or chronic substance abuse.

D. The treatment of amnesia can involve removing the agents contributing to the amnesia and helping the person develop memory aids.

IV. Mental disorders in later life

A. Mental disorders are less common among older adults than younger adults, but 10 to 20 percent of older people suffer significant psychopathology.

B. Psychological problems can be difficult to differentiate from medical problems. In addition, older people may complain of different symptoms than younger people do or may be less likely to seek help.

C. Anxiety disorders are fairly common among older people, particularly generalized anxiety disorder and posttraumatic stress disorder.

D. Anxiety disorders can be treated with antianxiety drugs, antidepressants, or psychotherapy.

E. Depression is a common problem among the elderly, and suicide rates are extremely high among elderly White males.

F. Some older people show a depletion syndrome, consisting of loss of interest, loss of energy, hopelessness, helplessness, and psychomotor retardation.

G. Differentiating depression from dementia can be particularly difficult, but certain patterns of memory loss can help in the differentiation.

H. Antidepressant medications and ECT are commonly used to treat severe depression in older people. Cognitive-behavioral and interpersonal therapies have been shown to work very well.

I. Alcohol use can become problematic as people age, particularly since the metabolism of and tolerance for alcohol change with age.

J. The abuse of and dependence on prescription drugs are significant problems among older people.

K. The treatment of substance use disorders for older people is similar to that for younger people.

KEY TERMS AND GUIDED REVIEW

cognitive disorders:

Guided Review

1. Why is the term "organic brain disorders" no longer used in DSM-IV-TR?

Dementia

Key Terms

dementia:

aphasia:

echolalia:

palialia:

apraxia:

agnosia:

executive functions:

Alzheimer's disease:

neurofibrillary tangles:

plaques:

amyloid:

vascular dementia:

cerebrovascular disease:

stroke:

Guided Review

1. How prevalent is Alzheimer's disease?

2. Describe each of the five types of cognitive deficits in dementia: memory impairment, aphasia, apraxia, agnosia, and deficits in executive functioning.

3. Describe some of the symptoms of Alzheimer's disease.

4. Describe the brain abnormalities in Alzheimer's disease. Where in the brain are these abnormalities concentrated?

5. Describe some of the proposed causes of Alzheimer's disease.

6. What is ApoE4? How is it related to Alzheimer's disease?

7. How are Alzheimer's disease and Down syndrome related?

8. Abnormalities on which chromosomes have been associated with increased risk of Alzheimer's disease?

9. Describe the neurotransmitter abnormalities in Alzheimer's disease.

10. How is vascular dementia different from Alzheimer's disease?

11. Among stroke patients, what factors are associated with increased risk of developing dementia?

12. What are some common causes of head injuries?

13. What is dementia pugilistica?

14. What is Parkinson's disease?

15. Describe the cognitive effects that can result from HIV.

16. What is Huntington's disease?

17. Describe the treatments that are available for dementia.

18. How does dementia vary by gender, ethnicity, and educational level?

Delirium

Key Terms

delirium:

Guided Review

1. Describe the symptoms of delirium.

2. Describe the onset of delirium.

3. What are some causes of delirium?

4. What are some risk factors for delirium?

5. What strategies are used to treat delirium?

Amnesia

<u>Key Terms</u>

amnesia:

anterograde amnesia:

retrograde amnesia:

<u>Guided Review</u>

1. What is the difference between anterograde and retrograde amnesia?

2. What are some causes of amnesia?

3. What is Korsakoff's syndrome?

4. What are some ways to treat amnesic disorders?

Mental Disorders in Later Life

<u>Key Term</u>

depletion syndrome:

<u>Guided Review</u>

1. Why can it be difficult to diagnose mental disorders (including depression and anxiety) among older adults?

2. Which anxiety disorders are common, and which are less common, among older adults?

3. What are some effective treatments for anxiety in older people?

4. What are some ways in which dementia and depression are similar? How can they be differentially diagnosed?

5. What are some effective treatments for depression in older people?

6. Describe how substance abuse tends to be manifested among older adults.

7. What are some characteristics of effective psychotherapies for older adults with substance abuse disorders?

CASE EXAMPLE
Read the following description and answer the questions below:

A 70-year-old college professor named Marshall has shown progressive deterioration in many areas of functioning over the last year. When he is alone in a store or in the woods near his home, he often gets lost and can't find his way out. He is easily distracted, and frequently forgets where he puts things. When this happens, Marshall often becomes angry and accuses others of taking his things. Marshall's wife has discovered a number of grave errors in his accounting in the family finances, such as major mathematical errors in the checkbook. When she has confronted him about these errors, Marshall has denied that there is anything wrong and has stomped off in a rage. Marshall's interest in his usual activities has diminished. He no longer wants to garden or read, when he formerly engaged in these activities almost daily. He is content to sit for long periods of time, or to shuffle and reshuffle the old letters and newspapers he has been collecting in his home office for the last couple of years. Conversations with Marshall can be difficult because he often uses odd words to refer to objects, such as calling a cup a vase, or goes on long tirades that are irrelevant to the subject being discussed. He does not seem to know anything that is going on in the world, although he sits in front of the television news programs every night. He recently asserted that John Kennedy was still president. Marshall has undergone extensive physical examinations in the past year, and no serious medical disease has been found. He has been only a light drinker of alcohol most of his life.

1. What cognitive disorder is Marshall most likely suffering from? What symptoms of this disorder does he show?

2. If Marshall's body undergoes an autopsy upon his death, what is likely to be found in his brain?

3. What treatments are available for Marshall's condition?

CHAPTER TEST

A. <u>Multiple Choice</u>. Choose the **best answer** to each question below.

1. By definition, a cognitive disorder cannot be caused by

    A. medical diseases.
    B. substance intoxication or withdrawal.

C. psychiatric disorders.

D. infections.

2. Dementia is

A. typically reversible with appropriate treatments.

B. caused by biological factors, whereas other disorders are not.

C. acute and usually transitory disorientation and memory loss.

D. gradual and usually permanent.

3. Which of the following is a term that refers to an impaired ability to execute common actions, such as waving goodbye?

A. Apraxia

B. Alogia

C. Agnosia

D. Aphasia

4. Which of the following would not be considered to reflect a deficit in executive functioning?

A. Interpreting the proverb, "People who live in glass houses shouldn't throw stones" to mean, "People don't want their windows broken."

B. Failing to recognize objects or people.

C. Difficulty planning how to carry out a sequence of actions.

D. Trouble stopping oneself from engaging in a behavior.

5. Repeating sounds or words over and over is known as

A. palialia.

B. aphasia.

C. echolalia.

D. apraxia.

6. The most common cause of dementia is ____.

A. stroke

B. Alzheimer's disease

C. brain injury

D. Parkinson's disease

7. Plaques are most likely to be found in the

A. precentral gyri.

B. occipital lobe.

C. hippocampus.

D. superior temporal lobe.

8. All of the following are pathological brain changes that occur in Alzheimer's disease except:

A. neurofibrillary tangles.
B. loss of dendrites.
C. shrunken ventricles.
D. extensive cell death.

9. Genetic abnormalities on which of the following chromosomes are associated with an increased risk of late-onset Alzheimer's disease?

A. 4
B. 14
C. 19
D. 21

10. Alzheimer's disease has been attributed to all of the following except:

A. viral infections.
B. excessive testosterone.
C. immune system dysfunction.
D. excessive aluminum.

11. Deficits in which of the following neurotransmitters are associated with declines in memory function in AD?

A. Peptide Y
B. Norepinephrine
C. Serotonin
D. Acetylcholine

12. All of the following are risk factors for the development of dementia in stroke patients except

A. having diabetes
B. being over the age of 80.
C. having a low level of education.
D. having arthritis.

13. All of the following are symptoms of frontal lobe injuries except

A. apathy.
B. uncharacteristic lewdness.
C. lability of affect.
D. visual-perceptual disturbances.

14. The most common causes of closed head injuries are

A. motor vehicle accidents.
B. falls.
C. gunshot wounds.
D. blows to the head during violent assaults.

15. Someone who experiences tremors, muscle rigidity, dementia, and inability to initiate movement would be most likely diagnosed with

    A. dementia pugilistica.
    B. Parkinson's disease.
    C. HIV-associated dementia.
    D. Huntington's disease.

16. Which of the following disorders is transmitted by a single dominant gene?

    A. Huntington's disease
    B. Parkinson's disease
    C. Alzheimer's disease
    D. Pick's disease

17. The nun study by Snowdon et al. (1996) showed that

    A. religious people are more likely to become demented.
    B. people who had greater linguistic skills earlier in life were less likely to develop Alzheimer's disease in late life.
    C. better-educated people were more likely to become demented because they had more abilities to lose once dementia took hold.
    D. people with low levels of education are less likely to be diagnosed with Alzheimer's disease than people with higher levels of education.

18. The diagnostic criteria for delirium include all of the following <u>except</u>:

    A. evidence that the disturbance is not caused by the direct physiological consequences of a medical condition.
    B. perceptual disturbance that is not accounted for by a dementia.
    C. reduced ability to focus, sustain, or shift attention.
    D. the disturbance develops over a short time and tends to fluctuate.

19. Korsakoff's syndrome is an amnestic disorder caused by damage to the _____.

    A. cerebral cortex
    B. amygdala
    C. thalamus
    D. hippocampus

20. Among people over 65

A. anxiety disorders are more prevalent among men than women.

B. approximately 20 percent can be diagnosed with a substance abuse disorder.

C. a first episode of bipolar disorder is quite common.

D. there is relatively no gender difference in rates of depression.

B. <u>True-False</u>. Select T (True) or F (False) below.

1. Dementia, delirium, and amnesia cannot be diagnosed if they appear to be the results of a psychiatric disorder, such as schizophrenia.   T   F

2. Individuals with higher levels of education are less likely to develop dementia. T   F

3. The degree of cognitive decline seen in Alzheimer's disease is significantly correlated with the degree of deficits in acetylcholine.   T   F

4. Antioxidants have been shown to slow cognitive decline in Alzheimer's disease. T   F

5. Parkinson's disease results from the death of cells that produce acetylcholine.   T   F

C. <u>Short Answer Questions</u>.

1. Describe the cognitive and biological deficits in Alzheimer's disease.

2. Describe several methods of distinguishing between depression and dementia.

3. What genetic factors are associated with increased risk of Alzheimer's disease?

4. Describe some ways in which dementia can be treated.

5. What is delirium? How is it similar to and different from dementia? How can it be treated?

ANSWER KEY

Case Example

1. Dementia of the Alzheimer's type. Memory impairment, impairment in abstract thinking, aphasia. This dementia is probably due to Alzheimer's because other illnesses that can cause dementia (e.g., Parkinson's disease, cerebrovascular disease, Huntington's disease, chronic alcoholism) have been ruled out.
2. Neurofibrillary plaques and tangles, cell death and dendritic shrinkage, enlarged ventricles, and neurotransmitter deficits.
3. Medications such as tacrine and donepezil, as well as antioxidants, ginkgo biloba, and anti-inflammatories. Behavior therapy may also be useful. None of these treatments will cure the disorder, but they may slow its progression or lead to slight improvement in symptoms.

Multiple Choice

1. C
2. D
3. A
4. B
5. A
6. B
7. C
8. C
9. C
10. B
11. D
12. D
13. D
14. A
15. B
16. A
17. B
18. A
19. C
20. D

True-False

1. T
2. T
3. T
4. T
5. F

Short Answer Questions

1. See pp. 515–518.
2. See p. 512.
3. See pp. 517–518.

4. See p. 522.
5. See pp. 525–527.

Additional Readings on Chapter 14 Topics

Bondi, M. W., Salmon, D. P., Galasko, D., Thomas, R. G., & Thal, L. J. (1999). Neuropsychological function and apolipoprotein E genotype in the preclinical detection of Alzheimer's disease. Psychology and Aging, 14, 295-303.

Grossman, M. (2002). Frontotemporal dementia: A review. Journal of the International Neuropsychological Society, 8, 566-583.

Parasuraman, R., Greenwood, P. M., & Sunderland, T. (2002). The apolipoprotein E gene, attention, and brain function. Neuropsychology, 16, 254-274.

Chapter 15: Eating Disorders

LEARNING OBJECTIVES

After reading and studying this chapter, you should be able to:

1. Discuss the gender similarities and differences in the eating disorders.

2. Discuss the key symptoms of anorexia nervosa, and distinguish between the restricting and the binge-purge type.

3. Discuss the prevalence of anorexia and its associated health risks.

4. Discuss the key symptoms of bulimia nervosa, and distinguish between the purging and nonpurging type.

5. Discuss the prevalence of bulimia and its associated health risks.

6. Identify the similarities and differences between anorexia and bulimia.

7. Discuss cultural and historical trends in the prevalence of eating disorders.

8. Discuss binge-eating disorder and how it differs from anorexia and bulimia.

9. Discuss the evidence that genetic factors contribute to the development of eating disorders.

10. Discuss the biological abnormalities in anorexia and bulimia.

11. Discuss the societal pressures on people (especially women) to maintain a slim appearance, and the behaviors people engage in to meet these expectations.

12. Discuss the impact of athletics on eating disorders.

13. Discuss the relationships among socioeconomic status, ethnicity, and eating disorders.

14. Discuss the emotional and cognitive styles of individuals with eating disorders.

15. Summarize the theories of Hilda Bruch and Salvador Minuchin.

16. Discuss the proposed explanations for why girls are at an increased risk for eating disorders compared to boys.

17. Discuss the argument that eating disorders result from sexual abuse, and summarize what the evidence suggests about this idea.

18. Discuss the difficulties faced by therapists who treat anorexic clients, and the ingredients of effective therapy for anorexia.

19. Discuss interpersonal, supportive-expressive, cognitive-behavioral, and behavioral therapies for bulimia, and their respective efficacy.

20. Describe how efficacious or inefficacious tricyclic antidepressants, MAO inhibitors, and selective serotonin reuptake inhibitors (SSRIs) are for treating anorexia and bulimia.

ESSENTIAL IDEAS

I. Anorexia nervosa

A. Anorexia nervosa is characterized by self-starvation, a distorted body image, intense fears of becoming fat, and amenorrhea.

B. People with the restricting type refuse to eat in order to prevent weight gain.

C. People with the binge/purge type periodically engage in bingeing and then purge to prevent weight gain.

D. The lifetime prevalence of anorexia is about 1 percent, with 90 to 95 percent of cases being female.

E. Anorexia usually begins in adolescence, and the course is variable from one person to another.

II. Bulimia nervosa

A. Bulimia nervosa is characterized by uncontrolled bingeing, followed by behaviors designed to prevent weight gain from the binges.

B. People with the purging type use self-induced vomiting, diuretics, or laxatives to prevent weight gain.

C. People with the nonpurging type use fasting and exercise to prevent weight gain.

D. The definition of a binge has been controversial, but the DSM-IV-TR specifies that it must involve the consumption of an unusually large amount of food in a short time, as well as a sense of lack of control.

E. The prevalence of the full syndrome of bulimia nervosa is estimated to be between 0.5 and 3 percent. It is much more common in women than in men.

F. The onset of bulimia nervosa is most often in adolescence, and its course, if left untreated, is unclear.

G. Although people with bulimia nervosa do not tend to be severely underweight, there are a variety of possible medical complications of the disorder.

III. Binge-eating disorder

A. Binge-eating disorder is a provisional diagnosis in the DSM-IV-TR. It is characterized by binge eating in the absence of behaviors designed to prevent weight gain.

B. Binge eating is common, perhaps more so among African Americans than among European Americans, but binge-eating disorder affects only about 2 percent of the population.

C. Women are more likely than men to develop binge-eating disorder.

IV. Understanding eating disorders

A. There is evidence that both anorexia nervosa and bulimia nervosa are heritable.

B. Eating disorders may be tied to dysfunction in the hypothalamus, a part of the brain that helps to regulate eating behavior.

C. Some studies show abnormalities in levels of the neurotransmitters serotonin and norepinephrine in people with eating disorders.

D. Cultural and societal norms regarding beauty may play a role in the eating disorders. Eating disorders are more common in groups that consider extreme thinness attractive than in groups that consider a heavier weight attractive.

E. Eating disorders develop as a means of gaining some control or of coping with negative emotions. In addition, people with eating disorders tend to show rigid, dichotomous thinking.

F. People who develop eating disorders tend to come from families that are overcontrolling and perfectionistic but that discourage the expression of negative emotions.

G. People who are so unaware of their own bodily sensations that they can starve themselves may develop anorexia nervosa. People who remain aware of their bodily sensations and cannot starve themselves but who are prone to anxiety and impulsivity may develop binge-eating disorder or bulimia nervosa.

H. Girls may be more likely than boys to develop eating disorders in adolescence because girls are not given as much freedom as boys to develop independence and their own identities.

I. People with eating disorders are more likely than people without eating disorders to have a history of sexual abuse, but a history of sexual abuse is also common among people with several other disorders.

V. Treatments for eating disorders

A. People with anorexia nervosa often must be hospitalized because they are so emaciated and malnourished that they are in a medical crisis.

B. Behavior therapy for anorexia nervosa involves making rewards contingent upon the client's eating. Clients may be taught relaxation techniques to handle their anxiety about eating.

C. Family therapy focuses on understanding the role of anorexic behaviors in the family unit. Therapists challenge parents' attitudes toward their children's behaviors and try to help the family find more adaptive ways of interacting with each other.

D. Individual therapy for anorexia may focus on helping clients identify and accept their feelings and to confront their distorted cognitions about their bodies.

E. Psychotherapy can be helpful for anorexia but is usually a long process, and the risk for relapse is high.

F. Several studies show that cognitive-behavioral therapy, which focuses on distorted cognitions about eating, is effective in the treatment of bulimia.

G. Interpersonal therapy, which focuses on the quality of a client's relationships, and supportive-expressive psychodynamic therapy, can be effective in the treatment of bulimia.

H. Tricyclic antidepressants and selective serotonin reuptake inhibitors have been shown to be helpful in the treatment of bulimia. The MAO inhibitors can also be helpful but are not usually prescribed because they require dietary restrictions to avoid side effects.

I. Antidepressants have not proven as useful in the treatment of anorexia nervosa, but some studies suggest the selective serotonin reuptake inhibitors may be helpful.

KEY TERMS AND GUIDED REVIEW

Guided Review

1. What are some of the gender differences in eating disorders?
Anorexia Nervosa

Key Terms

anorexia nervosa:

amenorrhea:

restricting type of anorexia nervosa:

binge/purge type of anorexia nervosa:

<u>Guided Review</u>

1. What are the symptoms of anorexia nervosa?

2. What are some differences between the restricting and binge/purge types of anorexia nervosa?

3. Describe the prevalence and course of anorexia nervosa.

4. What are some medical consequences of anorexia nervosa?

Bulimia Nervosa

<u>Key Terms</u>

bulimia nervosa:

bingeing:

purging type of bulimia nervosa:

nonpurging type of bulimia nervosa:

<u>Guided Review</u>

1. Describe some of the similarities and differences between anorexia and bulimia nervosa.

2. What are some of the differences between the purging and nonpurging types of bulimia nervosa?

3. Describe the prevalence and course of bulimia nervosa.

4. What are partial-syndrome eating disorders?

5. What are some medical consequences of bulimia?

6. Describe the evidence for cultural and historical differences in the prevalence of eating disorders.

Binge-Eating Disorder

<u>Key Term</u>

binge-eating disorder:

<u>Guided Review</u>

1. How is binge-eating disorder different from bulimia nervosa?

2. Among which groups is binge-eating disorder most common?

Understanding Eating Disorders

<u>Key Terms</u>

enmeshed families:

<u>Guided Review</u>

1. What is the evidence that eating disorders are influenced by genetics?

2. What are some biological contributors to eating disorders?

3. What are some of the societal pressures that may contribute to eating disorders?

4. Describe the relationship between athletics and eating disorders.

5. How do the eating disorders differ by socioeconomic status and ethnicity?

6. Describe the subtypes of disordered eating patterns identified by Stice and colleagues.

7. Describe the cognitive styles that are characteristic of individuals with eating disorders.

8. According to Hilde Bruch, how do family dynamics contribute to eating disorders?

9. What are some explanations for why eating disorders develop during adolescence and are more common among women?

10. What is the relationship between sexual abuse and eating disorders?

Treatments for Eating Disorders

<u>Guided Review</u>

1. Why are people with anorexia nervosa often difficult to treat?

2. Describe some of the methods used to treat individuals with anorexia nervosa in individual therapy.

3. Describe how family therapy for anorexia nervosa is conducted.

4. Describe some cognitive-behavioral techniques used to treat bulimia nervosa.

5. Describe some alternative types of therapy for bulimia nervosa. How effective are these types of therapy?

6. What treatments are effective for binge-eating disorder?

7. Which medications appear to be helpful for anorexia and bulimia nervosa?

CASE EXAMPLE
Read the following description and answer the questions below:

Tammy's family is just too perfect. Her parents are both very successful lawyers. Her older brother went to West Point and graduated at the top of his class. Her sister is a junior at an Ivy League college, carrying nearly a perfect grade point average, and has a great boyfriend. Tammy, on the other hand, is barely making it through high school, at least in her parents' eyes. She just can't seem to get her grades up to the standards set by her brother and sister. Her parents are constantly annoyed at her for not doing as well as they think she should. They have hired numerous tutors for Tammy, have transferred her to a private school (which she hates), and are constantly asking her about her exams and grades. They forbid her to date or even go out with friends much because they want her to spend all her time working on her grades and on "activities" that will help her get into a prestigious college. Tammy's parents don't have a lot of time for her, however. They both work about 80 hours a week and see Tammy mostly right before she goes to bed and for short periods on the weekend. Tammy seldom complains to her parents. She is grateful for any amount of time she can get with them and doesn't want to spoil it with conflict.

1. What characteristics of Tammy's family would Hilde Bruch and Salvador Minuchin say put Tammy at risk for an eating disorder?

2. If Tammy does develop an eating disorder, which of her characteristics might determine whether she develops anorexia or bulimia?

CHAPTER TEST

A. Multiple Choice. Choose the **best answer** to each question below.

1. Men who develop eating disorders

    A. display different symptoms of eating disorders than women.
    B. have high rates of comorbid substance abuse (like women), but do not have high rates of comorbid depression.
    C. are more likely than women to have a history of being overweight.
    D. are more likely than women to be athletes.

2. All of the following are diagnostic criteria for anorexia nervosa except:

    A. intense fear of gaining weight or becoming fat.
    B. absence of at least three menstrual cycles (in women who have reached menarche).
    C. refusal to maintain body weight at or above a minimally normal weight for one's age and height.
    D. recurrent episodes of binge eating.

3. Which of the following characterizes the binge/purge type of anorexia nervosa, but not the restricting type?

    A. Sense of lack of control over eating.
    B. Amenorrhea in females.
    C. Severely disturbed body image.
    D. Body weight at least 15 percent underweight.

4. Which of the following characterizes the binge/purge type of anorexia, but not bulimia nervosa?

    A. Binges, purges, or other compensatory behaviors.
    B. Body weight at least 15 percent underweight.
    C. Dissatisfaction with body size.
    D. Sense of lack of control over eating.

5. People with the restricting type of anorexia are more likely than those with the binge/purge type of anorexia

    A. to have problems with unstable moods.
    B. to have problems controlling their impulses.
    C. to have problems with self-mutilation.
    D. to have a deep mistrust of others and deny they have a problem.

6. The death rate among individuals with anorexia nervosa is approximately _____ percent.

A. 5
B. 15
C. 25
D. 35

7. Which of the following is <u>not</u> included in the DSM-IV-TR definition of a binge?

A. A binge includes a feeling of a lack of control over one's eating.
B. A binge must include a minimum of 1,500 calories.
C. A binge includes eating an amount of food that is definitely larger than most people would eat under similar circumstances.
D. A binge occurs in a discrete period of time.

8. All of the following are medical complications of anorexia nervosa <u>except</u>:

A. irregular heart rate.
B. tooth decay.
C. dehydration.
D. pancreatic disease.

9. People with which of the following eating disorders do <u>not</u> engage in binge eating?

A. Purging type of bulimia
B. Nonpurging type of bulimia
C. Binge-purge type of anorexia
D. Restricting type of anorexia

10. Which of the following is a known difference in the presentation of anorexia nervosa in Asian cultures, compared to American and European cultures?

A. Asians with anorexia nervosa are more preoccupied with being fat than Americans or Europeans with anorexia.
B. Asians with anorexia nervosa are more commonly restricted types, whereas more Americans and Europeans are binge/purge types.
C. Asians with anorexia nervosa do not have the distorted body images that are characteristic of American and European anorexia patients, and will often admit that they are thin.
D. More men than women have anorexia nervosa in Asian cultures.

11. Individuals with binge-eating disorder

A. often have memberships in weight-control programs.
B. are more commonly men than women.
C. are more commonly Asian American than African American.
D. are typically not dissatisfied with their bodies.

12. A brain area thought to be dysregulated in eating disorders is/are the

    A. hippocampus.
    B. thalamus.
    C. hypothalamus.
    D. parietal lobes.

13. Studies of bulimic people have found that they have abnormally low levels of

    A. norepinephrine.
    B. serotonin.
    C. acteylcholine.
    D. GABA.

14. Stice and colleagues found that body dissatisfaction in adolescent girls increased following

    A. their first date.
    B. a subscription to a fashion magazine.
    C. the onset of menstruation.
    D. their 15th birthday.

15. Eating disorders are more common among

    A. Hispanics.
    B. Caucasians.
    C. people of lower socioeconomic status.
    D. African Americans.

16. All of the following are characteristic thinking styles of people with eating disorders except

    A. a dichotomous thinking style in which everything is either all good or all bad.
    B. a tendency to highly value the opinions of others.
    C. the belief that one must be perfect.
    D. a tendency to blame oneself for other's failures.

17. The families of individuals with eating disorders can be characterized by all of the following except

    A. enmeshed.
    B. perfectionistic.
    C. permissive.
    D. overcontrolling.

18. Behavior therapies for anorexia

    A. have a low relapse rate.

B. benefit the majority of anorexic patients, who gain weight to within 15 percent of normal body weight.

C. are not an effective treatment for this disorder.

D. should involve the entire family.

19. Which of the following treatments has been shown to be most effective at reducing bingeing and purging among individuals with bulimia nervosa?

A. Dialectical behavior therapy
B. Interpersonal therapy
C. Supportive-expressive psychodynamic therapy
D. Cognitive-behavioral therapy

20. What types of medications are often effective in treating bulimia nervosa?

A. Antidepressants
B. Benzodiazepines
C. Antipsychotics
D. Mood stabilizers

B. <u>True-False</u>. Select T (True) or F (False) below.

1. The binge/purge type of anorexia is associated with a more chronic course of the disorder than the restricting type of anorexia.   T   F

2. People are more likely to die from bulimia than anorexia.   T   F

3. Tricyclic antidepressants and MAO inhibitors have not proven effective in the treatment of anorexia in controlled clinical trials.   T   F

4. People with eating disorders are more likely to have a history of sexual abuse than people with other psychological problems.   T   F

5. Individuals who participate in sports in which thinness is not emphasized have lower rates of eating disorders than non-athletes.   T   F

C. <u>Short Answer Questions</u>.

1. Describe the two types of anorexia and the two types of bulimia. How are these four disorders similar to and different from one another?

2. Describe Hilde Bruch's theory of anorexia nervosa.

3. What is the thin-ideal, where does it come from, and what effect does it have on girls and women?

4. What treatments are effective for anorexia and bulimia nervosa?

5. Describe some biological contributors to the eating disorders.

ANSWER KEY

Case Example
1. "Perfectionism in family"; parents overcontrolling but uninvolved emotionally; chronic tension between Tammy and her parents, which is not openly expressed.
2. If Tammy is able to ignore or is unable to read her body's signals about hunger, she is more likely to develop restricting anorexia. If she finds that binge-eating helps to relieve her negative emotions, she is more likely to develop bulimia.

Multiple Choice
1. C
2. D
3. A
4. B
5. D
6. A
7. B
8. D
9. D
10. C
11. A
12. C
13. A
14. B
15. B
16. D
17. C
18. B
19. D
20. A

True-False
1. T
2. F
3. T
4. F
5. T

Short Answer Questions
1. See pp. 545–548.
2. See pp.559–561.
3. See pp.554–556.
4. See pp. 562–567.
5. See pp. 553–554.

Additional Readings on Chapter 15 Topics

Dingemans, A. E., Bruna, M. J., & van Furth, E. F. (2002). Binge eating disorder: A review. International Journal of Obesity and Related Metabolic Disorders, 26, 299-307.

Fairburn, C. G., Shafran, R., & Cooper, Z. (1999). A cognitive behavioural theory of anorexia nervosa. Behaviour Research and Therapy, 37, 1-13.

Wilson, G. T., Fairburn, C. C., Agras, W. S., Walsh, B. T., & Kraemer, H. (2002). Cognitive-behavioral therapy for bulimia nervosa: Time course and mechanisms of change. Journal of Consulting and Clinical Psychology, 70, 267-274.

Chapter 16: Sexual Disorders

LEARNING OBJECTIVES

After reading and studying this chapter, you should be able to:

1. Describe the five stages of the sexual response cycle, and the gender differences evident in it.

2. Distinguish between hypoactive sexual desire and sexual aversion disorder.

3. Describe female sexual arousal disorder and male erectile disorder.

4. Describe female orgasmic disorder (anorgasmia), male orgasmic disorder, and premature ejaculation.

5. Describe dyspareunia and vaginismus.

6. Discuss the biological causes of sexual dysfunctions, including specific medical conditions and drugs, and how biologically-caused dysfunctions differ from those caused by psychological factors.0-p

7. Discuss the relationship problems, traumas, and attitudes that can cause sexual dysfunctions.

8. Discuss some cultural differences in sexual dysfunctions.

9. Discuss age-related changes that can impact sexual functioning.

10. Discuss the drugs and biological procedures used to treat sexual dysfunctions.

11. Describe how couples therapy and individual psychotherapy can be useful to treat sexual dysfunctions.

12. Discuss components of sex therapy, such as sensate focus therapy, the stop-start technique, and the squeeze technique.

13. Describe issues that are unique to gay, lesbian, and bisexual individuals suffering from sexual dysfunctions.

14. Discuss the differences between paraphilias and normal sexual fantasies.

15. Describe fetishism, sexual sadism, sexual masochism, voyeurism, exhibitionism, and frotteurism.

16. Discuss the causes, characteristics, and available treatments for pedophilia.

17. Distinguish among gender identity, gender role, and sexual orientation.

18. Discuss the characteristics of and treatments for gender identity disorder.

19. Distinguish between transsexualism and transvestitism.

ESSENTIAL IDEAS

I. Sexual dysfunctions

A. The sexual response cycle includes five phases: desire, excitement or arousal, plateau, orgasm, and resolution.

B. People with disorders of sexual desire have little or no desire to engage in sex. These disorders include hypoactive sexual desire disorder and sexual aversion disorder.

C. People with sexual arousal disorders do not experience the physiological changes that make up the excitement or arousal phase of the sexual response cycle. These disorders include female sexual arousal disorder and male erectile disorder.

D. Women with female orgasmic disorder do not experience orgasm or have greatly delayed orgasm after reaching the excitement phase. Men with premature ejaculation reach ejaculation before they wish to. Men with male orgasmic disorder have a recurrent delay in or absence of orgasm following sexual excitement.

E. The two sexual pain disorders are dyspareunia, genital pain associated with intercourse, and vaginismus, involuntary contraction of the vaginal muscles in women.

F. The biological causes of sexual dysfunctions include undiagnosed diabetes or other medical conditions, prescription or recreational drug use (including alcohol), and hormonal or vascular abnormalities.

G. The psychological causes include psychological disorders and maladaptive attitudes and cognitions (especially performance concerns).

H. The sociocultural and interpersonal causes include problems in intimate relationships, traumatic experiences, and an upbringing or cultural environment that devalues or degrades sex.

I. When the cause of a sexual dysfunction is biological, treatments that eradicate the cause can cure the sexual dysfunction. Alternately, drug therapies or prostheses can be used.

J. Sex therapy corrects the inadequate sexual practices of a client and his or her partner. The techniques of sex therapy include sensate focus therapy, instruction in masturbation, the stop-start and squeeze techniques, and the deconditioning of vaginal contractions.

K. Couples therapy focuses on decreasing conflicts between couples over their sexual practices or over other areas of their relationship.

L. Individual psychotherapy helps people recognize conflicts or negative attitudes behind their sexual dysfunctions and resolve these.

II. Paraphilias

A. The paraphilias are a group of disorders in which people's sexual activity is focused on (1) nonhuman objects, (2) nonconsenting adults, (3) suffering or the humiliation of oneself or one's partner, or (4) children.

B. Fetishism involves the use of inanimate objects (such as panties or shoes) as the preferred or exclusive source of sexual arousal or gratification. One elaborate fetish is transvestism, in which a man dresses in the clothes of a woman to sexually arouse himself.

C. Voyeurism involves observing another person nude or engaging in sexual acts, without that person's knowledge or consent, in order to become sexually aroused.

D. Exhibitionism involves exposing oneself to another without that person's consent, in order to become sexually aroused.

E. Frotteurism involves rubbing up against another without his or her consent, in order to become sexually aroused.

F. Sadism and masochism involve physically harming another or allowing oneself to be harmed for sexual arousal.

G. Pedophilia involves engaging in sexual acts with a child.

H. Behavioral theories suggest that the sexual behaviors of people with paraphilias results from classical and operant conditioning.

I. Treatments for the paraphilias include biological interventions to reduce sexual drive, behavioral interventions to decondition arousal to paraphillic objects, and training in interpersonal and social skills.

III. Gender identity disorder

A. Gender identity disorder (GID) is diagnosed when individuals believe they were born with the wrong sex's genitals and are fundamentally persons of the opposite sex. This disorder in adults is also called transsexualism.

B. Biological theories suggest that unusual exposure to prenatal hormones affects the development of the hypothalamus and other brain structures involved in sexuality, leading to gender identity disorder.

C. Socialization theories suggest that the parents of children (primarily boys) with gender identity disorder do not socialize gender-appropriate behaviors. Other theories suggest that the parents of children who develop this disorder have high rates of psychopathology.

D. Some people with this disorder undergo gender reassignment treatment to change their genitalia and live as a member of the sex they believe they are.

KEY TERMS AND GUIDED REVIEW

Sexual Dysfunctions

<u>Key Terms</u>

sexual dysfunctions:

sexual desire:

arousal phase:

vasocongestion:

myotonia:

plateau phase:

orgasm:

resolution:

hypoactive sexual desire disorder:

sexual aversion disorder:

female sexual arousal disorder:

male erectile disorder:

female orgasmic disorder:

premature ejaculation:

male orgasmic disorder:

dyspareunia:

vaginismus:

substance-induced sexual dysfunction:

performance anxiety:

sensate focus therapy:

stop-start technique:

squeeze technique:

Guided Review

1. Define each of the five stages of the sexual response cycle.

2. Describe some of the differences between male and female sexual responses.

3. Why are more people seeking sex therapy?

4. What is the difference between a generalized and situational sexual desire disorder?

5. How does hypoactive sexual desire differ by gender?

6. What is the difference between the lifelong and acquired forms of male erectile disorder?

7. What are the criteria for female orgasmic disorder?

8. How do premature ejaculation and male orgasmic disorder differ?

9. Describe how dyspareunia is manifested in both men and women.

10. What are some areas that a clinician should assess when he or she suspects a sexual dysfunction?

11. What are some common medical causes of sexual dysfunction?

12. What is the relationship between hormones and sexual functioning in men and women?

13. Give some examples of drugs that can affect sexual functioning.

14. What are some differences between biologically and psychologically caused sexual dysfunctions?

15. Give some examples of psychological disorders and attitudes or cognitions that can interfere with sexual functioning.

16. Describe some ways in which men gain ejaculatory control.

17. Give some examples of how problems in relationships (e.g., communication difficulties) can lead to sexual dysfunctions.

18. What are some ways in which trauma can lead to sexual dysfunctions?

19. Give some examples of cross-cultural differences in sexual behavior or sexual dysfunctions.

20. Describe some age-related changes that can affect sexual functioning.

21. Describe some of the biological treatments available for sexual dysfunctions.

22. What are some issues addressed in couple or individual psychotherapy for sexual dysfunctions?

23. What are the elements of sensate focus therapy?

24. Give an example of how (1) premature ejaculation and (2) vaginismus may be treated.

25. What are some special issues faced by gay, lesbian, and bisexual people with respect to sexual functioning?

26. Give some examples of folk remedies for sexual dysfunctions.

Paraphilias

Key Terms

paraphilias:

fetishism:

transvestism:

sexual sadism:

sexual masochism:

sadomasochism:

voyeurism:

exhibitionism:

frotteurism:

pedophilia:

aversion therapy:

desensitization:

Guided Review

1. What are some characteristics of people with paraphilias?

2. Give some examples of fetishes.

3. Why do some clinicians question if fetishism should qualify as a psychiatric diagnosis?

4. What are the sources of sexual excitement in sadomasochism, voyeurism, exhibitionism, and frotteurism?

5. What are the criteria for a diagnosis of pedophilia?

6. What are some effects of child sexual abuse?

7. What are the psychodynamic, behavioral, social learning, and cognitive theories of paraphilias?

8. Describe some of the effective treatments for paraphilias.

Gender Identity Disorder

Key Terms

gender identity:

gender role:

sexual orientation:

gender identity disorder (GID):

transsexuals:

1. How do the terms gender identity, gender role, and sexual orientation differ from one another?

2. What are the criteria for gender identity disorder?

3. How does transsexualism differ from transvestism?

4. What are some biological contributors to gender identity disorder?

5. How might parents contribute to the development of gender identity disorder in their children?

6. Describe gender reassignment and its advantages and disadvantages.

CASE EXAMPLE

Read the following description and answer the questions below:

Alan and Kim have requested couples therapy because their "sex life has all but ended." For the past several months, whenever they have tried to have sex together, Alan has not been able to sustain an erection and Kim has not had an orgasm. They now report that neither of them has much interest in having sex with the other. Their problems began after Alan started a new job that he finds highly stressful and tiring. He works 6 to 7 days a week every week. He comes home each night at 8 or 9 P.M., exhausted. When Kim tries to talk with him about the events of the day, he recounts all the disagreements he had with people on the job, and how frustrated he is. He doesn't listen when Kim tries to tell him about her own day. Kim's response to this has been to withdraw, to do dishes while Alan watches television and falls asleep. Kim has also begun to have "dates" with a man she works with. These dates started as casual lunches during the work day. But when Alan is on a business trip, Kim has dinner with this man, and once she kissed this man passionately at the end of one of these dates. Kim feels badly about "cheating" on Alan and wants to maintain her marriage. Alan knows his marriage is in trouble, and he also wants to save it.

1. What diagnoses, if any, do Alan's and Kim's behaviors and feelings warrant?

2. What might be an effective course of therapy for Alan and Kim?

CHAPTER TEST

A. <u>Multiple Choice</u>. Choose the **best answer** to each question below.

1. Which of the following is <u>not</u> one of Masters and Johnson's five phases of the sexual response cycle?

    A. Resolution
    B. Arousal
    C. Orgasm
    D. Refractory period

2. Enlargement of the clitoris, swelling of the labia, and moistening of the vagina is caused by

    A. myotonia.
    B. engorgement.
    C. orgasm.
    D. the refractory period.

3. During the _____ phase, vasocongestion and myotonia occur.

    A. desire
    B. orgasm
    C. arousal
    D. plateau

4. Recurrent inability to attain or maintain the swelling-lubrication response of sexual excitement is known as

    A. sexual aversion disorder.
    B. female orgasmic disorder.
    C. female sexual arousal disorder.
    D. vaginismus.

5. The most common complaint of people seeking sex therapy is

    A. lack of sexual desire.
    B. inability to experience orgasm.
    C. pain or discomfort during sex.
    D. difficulty staying sexually aroused.

6. Genital pain associated with sexual intercourse is known as

    A. hypoactive sexual desire disorder.
    B. dyspareunia.
    C. vaginismus.

D. sexual aversion disorder.

7. Hypoactive sexual desire disorder is

   A. diagnosed only in individuals who have never enjoyed sex.
   B. diagnosed when low sexual desire results from pain during intercourse.
   C. more common in older women and younger men.
   D. more often connected to anxiety or depression in women than in men.

8. The most common orgasmic disorder in men is

   A. premature ejaculation.
   B. male orgasmic disorder.
   C. male erectile disorder.
   D. dyspareunia.

9. Which of the following statements about the causes of sexual dysfunction is <u>true</u>?

   A. In men, low levels of prolactin and estrogen can cause sexual dysfunctions.
   B. In women, hormones have a consistent, direct effect on sexual desire.
   C. Psychologically caused sexual dysfunctions tend to be global and consistent.
   D. Early masturbation practices can lead to sexual difficulties in adulthood.

10. "Spectatoring" involves

   A. voyeurs watching people engaged in sex without the people's consent or awareness.
   B. exhibitionists revealing themselves to large groups of people at the same time.
   C. individuals closely monitoring their own behaviors and feelings while engaging in sexual relations with another person.
   D. parents allowing their children to watch them engage in sexual intercourse.

11. Men gain ejaculatory control through all of the following processes <u>except</u>:

   A. a regular rhythm of being sexual.
   B. adherence to the same intercourse position.
   C. increased comfort with practice.
   D. a more give-and-take pleasuring process.

12. Men seeking treatment for hypoactive sexual desire disorder are more likely than women

   A. to report problems in their marriage.
   B. to be experiencing other types of sexual dysfunction.
   C. to report other stressful events in their lives.
   D. to have higher levels of psychological distress.

13. The traditional Chinese medical system teaches that

A. loss of semen is detrimental to a man's health.

B. if a man does not have an erection, then he does not want sex.

C. pregnancy is more likely when women's vaginas are dry and tight for sexual intercourse.

D. masturbation has very positive effects on one's health.

14. The stop-start technique is used primarily

A. to help a paraphilic stop engaging in paraphilic behavior and start engaging in normal sexual behavior.

B. to help men who have premature ejaculations learn to control their ejaculations.

C. to help women with vaginismus gain some control over their vaginal contractions.

D. to help women with dyspareunia learn they can stop sexual interactions when they feel pain and start them again when the pain passes.

15. Someone who obtains sexual arousal by compulsively and secretly watching another person being naked or engaging in sex would most likely be diagnosed with

A. exhibitionism.

B. frotteurism.

C. voyeurism.

D. fetishism.

16. Someone who obtains sexual gratification from stealing women's underwear and masturbating into them would most likely be diagnosed with

A. fetishism.

B. transsexualism.

C. transvestism.

D. exhibitionism.

17. All of the following statements are true about pedophiles except:

A. pedophiles have typically been abused as children.

B. pedophiles are typically homosexual.

C. the typical victims of pedophiles are relatives or close acquaintances.

D. pedophiles must be, by definition, at least 5 years older than their victim(s).

18. Drugs that reduce sexual drive and are used to treat sex offenders include

A. calcium channel blockers.

B. benzodiazepines.

C. selective serotonin reuptake inhibitors (SSRIs).

D. testosterone.

19. Which of the following statements is true regarding the treatment of sex offenders?

A. Treatment outcome studies reveal that treatment has no effect on the reduction of sexual offenses.
B. Rapists respond the best to cognitive therapy.
C. Medications are not effective at reducing paraphilic behavior.
D. Treatment outcome studies show that psychosocial interventions reduce sexual offenses.

20. All of the following are criteria for gender identity disorder except

A. intense desire to participate in the stereotypical games and pastimes of the other sex.
B. strong preference for playmates of the other sex.
C. repeatedly stated desire to be, or insistence that he or she is, the other sex.
D. evidence of prenatal hormonal abnormalities is present.

B. <u>True-False</u>. Select T (True) or F (False) below.

1. In most cases of hypoactive sexual desire, the individual has never had much interest in sex.
   T   F

2. Most pedophiles are homosexual men abusing young boys.   T   F

3. In transsexualism, people dress as a member of the opposite gender in order to gain sexual satisfaction.   T   F

4. Viagra and other drugs that are used to treat male erectile disorder are not effective if the erectile dysfunction is caused by a medical problem.   T   F

5. Early versions of the DSM listed homosexuality as a mental disorder.   T   F

C. <u>Short Answer Questions</u>.

1. What are some special considerations that should be made when treating gay men and lesbians with sexual dysfunction?

2. Identify and describe the five phases of the sexual response cycle as it occurs in both men and women.

3. Describe the process of sensate focus therapy.

4. Describe the behavioral and social-learning theories of paraphilias.

5. What are some of the proposed explanations for gender identity disorder?

ANSWER KEY

<u>Case Example</u>
1. Male erectile disorder for Alan and female orgasmic disorder for Kim. Hypoactive sexual desire would not be diagnosed for either of them because it is secondary to the primary disorders.
2. Couples therapy focusing on couple's "seduction rituals" and on the communication patterns between Alan and Kim. If Kim reveals her dating of another man, therapy will need to deal with Alan's reactions to this and whether the couple is committed enough to the relationship to learn to ask for what they need from each other and to give what each other needs.

<u>Multiple Choice</u>
1. D
2. B
3. C
4. C
5. A
6. B
7. D
8. A
9. D
10. C
11. B
12. B
13. A
14. B
15. C
16. A
17. B
18. C
19. D
20. D

<u>True-False</u>
1. F
2. F
3. F
4. F
5. T

<u>Short Answer Questions</u>
1. See p. 597.
2. See pp. 576–578.
3. See pp. 594–595.
4. See p. 604.
5. See pp. 610–611.

Additional Readings on Chapter 16 Topics

Haldeman, D. C. (2002). Gay rights, patient rights: The implications of sexual orientation conversion therapy. Professional Psychology: Research and Practice, 33, 260-264.

Scholinski, D. (1998). The last time I wore a dress. New York: Riverhead Books. *This is a fascinating story about gender identity disorder.*

Wilson, I., Griffin, C., & Wren, B. (2002). The validity of the diagnosis of gender identity disorder (child and adolescent criteria). Clinical Child Psychology and Psychiatry, 7, 335-351.

Chapter 17: Substance-Related Disorders

LEARNING OBJECTIVES

After reading and studying this chapter, you should be able to:

1. Discuss the prevalence, patterns, and trends of substance use over the past several decades, and how the rates of substance use vary by culture, gender, and age.

2. Distinguish among and define substance intoxication, withdrawal, abuse, and dependence, and the factors associated with different manifestations of intoxication, withdrawal, and dependence.

3. Describe the intoxication and withdrawal effects (when such effects exist) of alcohol, benzodiazepines, barbiturates, inhalants, cocaine, amphetamines, nicotine, caffeine, opioids, hallucinogens, PCP, cannabis, ecstasy, GHB, ketamine, and rohypnol.

4. Discuss the negative effects of the substances described in this chapter on physical and mental health.

5. Describe the stages of alcohol withdrawal.

6. Discuss the typical patterns of alcohol, benzodiazepine, barbiturate, and cocaine use that lead to dependence on these substances.

7. Define and describe Wernicke's encephalopathy, Korsakoff's psychosis, alcohol-induced dementia, and fetal alcohol syndrome.

8. Distinguish between the disease model of alcoholism and the controlled drinking perspective.

9. Summarize the contributions of dopamine neurons in the "pleasure pathway" to substance use behavior.

10. Discuss the role of genetics in alcoholism and describe what might be inherited by the children of alcoholics.

11. Summarize the arguments and evidence for and against the idea that alcoholism is a form of depression.

12. Discuss the appropriate uses of methadone, naltrexone, naloxone, disulfiram, and antidepressants to treat people with particular substance-related disorders.

13. Describe Alcoholics Anonymous and its treatment philosophy.

14. Discuss the behavioral treatments for alcoholism: aversive classical conditioning, covert sensitization therapy, and cue exposure and response prevention.

15. Describe the elements of behavioral and cognitive therapies for alcoholism, and the elements of relapse prevention programs.

16. Discuss why different treatment approaches may be indicated for men and women.

ESSENTIAL IDEAS

I. Society and substance use

A. Cultures differ in their predominant attitudes and legal policies regarding substances. Many Muslim countries strictly prohibit alcohol. The British consider substance addiction to be a medical disease, and refer most users for treatment rather than punishment. The Dutch distinguish "hard" drugs (such as heroin) from "soft" drugs (such as cannabis) and only aggressively prosecute the use and sale of "hard" drugs in an attempt to avoid driving users of "soft" drugs underground where they might begin using more potent substances.

B. Many substances, including stimulants, opioids, and hallucinogens, have been used by various cultures throughout history for medicinal or religious purposes. People who deliberately use substances to alter their moods, thoughts, and behaviors as ends in themselves and who experience significant distress and/or impairment in their daily functioning are said to have a substance-related disorder.

II. Defining substance-related disorders

A. Substance intoxication is a set of behavioral and psychological changes that result directly from the physiological effects of a substance on the central nervous system.

B. Substance withdrawal is a set of physiological and behavioral symptoms that result from a reduction or cessation of substance use following a prolonged period of heavy use. Withdrawal symptoms are typically the opposite of symptoms experienced during intoxication and tend to begin and end more quickly for substances that quickly exit the body, and more slowly for substances that slowly exit the body.

C. Substance abuse is diagnosed when an individual experiences recurrent problems in at least one of the following four areas over a 12-month period: (1) failure to fulfill important obligations at work, school, or home; (2) use of substances in physically hazardous situations; (3) legal problems as a result of substance use; and (4) recurrent substance use despite significant social or legal problems that result from the substance use.

D. Substance dependence is diagnosed when a person compulsively uses a substance despite significant social, occupational, psychological, or medical problems as a result of the use. Substances vary in their potential to lead to dependence: those that are rapidly and efficiently absorbed (e.g., by injection), that act more rapidly on the central nervous system, that cause intoxication quickly, and whose effects wear off quickly, are most likely to lead to dependence.

III. Depressants

A. At low doses, alcohol produces relaxation and a mild euphoria. At higher doses, it produces the classic signs of depression and cognitive and motor impairment.

B. A large proportion of deaths due to accidents, murders, and suicides are alcohol-related.

C. Alcohol withdrawal symptoms can be mild or so severe as to be life threatening.

D. People who abuse alcohol or are dependent on alcohol experience a wide range of social and interpersonal problems and are at risk for many serious health problems.

E. Women drink less alcohol than do men in most cultures and are less likely to have alcohol-related disorders than are men.

F. Benzodiazepines and barbiturates are sold legally by prescription for the treatment of anxiety and insomnia.

G. Benzodiazepines and barbiturates can cause an initial rush plus a loss of inhibitions. These pleasurable sensations are then followed by depressed mood, lethargy, and physical signs of central nervous system depression.

H. Benzodiazepines and barbiturates are dangerous in overdose and when mixed with other substances.

I. Inhalants are substances that produce chemical vapors, such as gasoline or paint thinner. Inhalants can cause permanent organ and brain damage and accidental deaths due to suffocation or dangerous delusional behavior.

IV. Stimulants

A. Cocaine and the amphetamines produce a rush of euphoria, followed by increases in self-esteem, alertness, and energy. With chronic use, however, they can lead to grandiosity, impulsiveness, hypersexuality, agitation, and paranoia.

B. Withdrawal from cocaine and the amphetamines causes symptoms of depression, exhaustion, and an intense craving for more of the substances.

C. Cocaine seems particularly prone to lead to dependence, because it has extraordinarily rapid and strong effects on the brain and its effects wear off quickly.

D. The intense activation of the central nervous system caused by cocaine and the amphetamines can lead to a number of cardiac, respiratory, and neurological problems, and these substances are responsible for a large percentage of substance-related medical emergencies and deaths.

E. Nicotine is an alkaloid found in tobacco. It affects the release of several neurochemicals in the body. Nicotine subjectively reduces stress but causes physiological arousal similar to that seen in the fight-or-flight response.

F. Smoking is associated with a higher rate of heart disease, lung cancer, emphysema, and chronic bronchitis, and it substantially increases mortality rates.

G. The majority of people who smoke wish they could quit, but have trouble doing so, in part because tolerance develops to nicotine and withdrawal symptoms are difficult to tolerate.

H. Caffeine is the most commonly used stimulant drug. Caffeine intoxication can cause agitation, tremors, heart irregularities, and insomnia. People can develop a tolerance for and withdrawal from caffeine.

V. Opioids

A. The opioids include heroin, morphine, codeine, and methadone, and synthetic opioids include hydrocodone (Lorcet, Lortab, Vicodin) and oxycodone (Percodan, Percocet, Oxycontin).

B. The opioids cause an initial rush, or euphoria, followed by a drowsy, dream-like state. Severe intoxication can cause respiratory and cardiovascular failure.

C. Withdrawal symptoms include dysphoria, anxiety, and agitation; an achy feeling in the back and legs; increased sensitivity to pain; and craving for more opioids.

D. Opioid users who inject drugs can contract HIV and a number of other diseases by sharing needles.

VI. Hallucinogens and PCP

A. The hallucinogens create perceptual illusions and distortions, sometimes fantastic, sometimes frightening. They cause some people to feel more sensitive to art, music, and other people. They also create mood swings and paranoia. Some people experience frightening flashbacks to experiences under the hallucinogens.

B. PCP causes euphoria or affective dulling, abnormal involuntary movements, and weakness at low doses. At intermediate doses, it leads to disorganized thinking, depersonalization, feelings of unreality, and aggression. At higher doses, it produces amnesia and coma, analgesia sufficient to allow surgery, seizures, severe respiratory problems, hypothermia, and hyperthermia.

VII. Cannabis

A. Cannabis creates a high feeling, cognitive and motor impairments, and in some people, hallucinogenic effects.

B. Cannabis use is high. Significant numbers of people, especially teenagers, have impaired performance at school, on the job, and in relationships as a result of chronic use. Marijuana use can also lead to a number of physical problems, especially respiratory problems.

VIII. Club drugs

A. Some common club drugs, in addition to LSD, are ecstasy (3-4 methylenedioxymethamphetamine, or MDMA), GHB (gamma-hydroxybutyrate), ketamine, and rohypnol (flunitrazepam).

B. Ecstasy has the stimulant effects of an amphetamine along with occasional hallucinogenic properties. Even short-term use of ecstasy can have long-term negative effects on cognition and health. Long-term users of ecstasy are at risk for several cardiac problems and liver failure, and they show increased rates of anxiety, depression, psychotic symptoms, and paranoia.

C. GHB is an anabolic steroid and a central nervous system depressant. At low doses it can relieve anxiety and promote relaxation. At higher doses, it can result in sleep, coma, or death.

D. Ketamine is an anesthetic that produces hallucinogenic effects. Large doses can produce vomiting and convulsions, and even death.

E. Rohypnol has sedative and hypnotic effects. It is one of the date rape drugs, along with GHB and ketamine. When used in combination with alcohol or other depressants, it can be fatal.

IX. Theories of substance use, abuse, and dependence

A. Psychoactive substances have powerful effects on the parts of the brain that register reward and pleasure. The repeated use of a substance may sensitize this system, causing a craving for more of the substance.

B. Substance use disorders appear to be influenced by genetics. The genes involved in these disorders influence neurotransmitters that regulate the metabolism and biosynthesis of substances.

C. Some theorists view alcoholism as a form of depression, although the prevailing evidence suggests that alcoholism and depression are distinct disorders.

D. Behavioral theories of alcoholism note that people are reinforced or punished by other people for their alcohol-related behaviors and model alcohol-related behaviors from parents and important others.

E. Cognitive theories argue that people who develop alcohol-related problems have strong expectations that alcohol will help them feel better and cope better when they face stressful times.

F. One personality trait associated with increased risk for substance use disorders is behavioral undercontrol, which, in turn, appears to be influenced by genetics.

G. Sociocultural theorists note that alcohol and drug use increases among people under severe stress.

H. In addition, the gender differences in substance-related disorders may be due to men having more risk factors for substance use and women being more sensitive to the negative consequences of substance use.

X. Treatments for substance-related disorders

A. Detoxification is the first step in treating substance-related disorders.

B. Antianxiety and antidepressant drugs can help ease withdrawal symptoms. Antagonist drugs can block the effects of substances, reducing desire for the drug, or making the ingestion of the drug aversive.

C. Methadone maintenance programs substitute methadone for heroin in the treatment of heroin addicts. These programs are controversial but may be the only way to help some heroin addicts withdraw from heroin.

D. Behavioral therapies based on aversive classical conditioning are sometimes used to treat substance use disorders.

E. Treatments based on social learning and cognitive theories focus on training people with substance use disorders in more adaptive coping skills and challenging their positive expectations about the effects of substances.

F. The most common treatment for alcoholism is Alcoholics Anonymous, a self-help group that encourages alcoholics to admit their weaknesses and to call on a higher power and other group members to help them remain completely abstinent from alcohol. Related groups are available for people dependent on other substances.

G. Prevention programs for college students aim to teach them responsible use of alcohol.

H. Different treatments may be needed for men and women that take into account the different contexts for their substance use.

KEY TERMS AND GUIDED REVIEW

<u>Key Terms</u>

substance:

drug addicts:

<u>Guided Review</u>

1. Describe patterns of substance use in the United States, and highlight differences in substance use by gender and ethnicity.

Society and Substance Use

<u>Key Terms</u>

substance-related disorder:

<u>Guided Review</u>

1. Give some examples of how different societies view substance use.

2. What are some reasons that societies may want to regulate substance use?

Defining Substance-Related Disorders

<u>Key Terms</u>

substance intoxication:

substance withdrawal:

substance abuse:

substance dependence:

tolerance:

<u>Guided Review</u>

1. What is substance intoxication? Under what circumstances is it diagnosed?

2. The symptoms of intoxication depend on which factors?

3. What is substance withdrawal? When is it diagnosed?

4. What is substance abuse? What must be present for it to be diagnosed?

5. What is substance dependence?

6. What is physiological dependence?

7. Why is the route of administration used to ingest a substance important?

Depressants

Key Terms

blackout:

alcohol abuse:

alcohol dependence:

delirium tremens (DTs):

alcohol-induced persisting amnestic disorder:

Wernicke's encephalopathy:

Korsakoff's psychosis:

alcohol-induced dementia:

fetal alcohol syndrome (FAS):

benzodiazepines:

barbiturates:

inhalants:

Guided Review

1. What are some of the intoxication and withdrawal effects of depressants?

2. How are alcohol abuse and dependence different from one another?

3. Describe the patterns of alcohol use by alcohol abusers and dependents.

4. How do alcoholics with antisocial personalities differ from alcoholics without antisocial personalities?

5. What is negative affect alcoholism?

6. Describe the stages of alcohol withdrawal.

7. What are some of the long-term health effects of alcohol abuse?

8. Identify and describe some of the neurological disorders that can result from alcohol abuse.

9. Describe some cross-cultural differences in alcohol abuse and dependence.

10. How do the rates of alcohol problems vary by age and gender?

11. What are the common patterns in the development of benzodiazepine or barbiturate abuse and dependence?

12. What are some negative effects of inhalant abuse?

Stimulants

<u>Key Terms</u>

cocaine:

amphetamines:

nicotine:

caffeine:

<u>Guided Review</u>

1. Describe some of the intoxication and withdrawal effects of stimulants.

2. Why is cocaine more likely than other substances to result in patterns of substance abuse and dependence?

3. What happens in the brain after someone ingests cocaine?

4. Describe some of the negative consequences of amphetamine abuse.

5. Describe the physiological effects of nicotine.

6. Describe the negative health effects of smoking.

7. What is the evidence that nicotine is addictive?

8. Describe the physiological effects of caffeine.

9. What are the symptoms of caffeine intoxication?

Opioids

<u>Key Term</u>

opioids:

<u>Guided Review</u>

1. What are some of the intoxication and withdrawal effects of opioids?

2. Describe some negative health and psychosocial effects of opioids.

Hallucinogens and PCP

<u>Key Terms</u>

hallucinogens:

phenylcyclidine (PCP):

<u>Guided Review</u>

1. Describe the intoxication effects of hallucinogens and PCP.

2. What are some negative mental and physical health effects of PCP?

Cannabis

<u>Key Term</u>

cannabis:

<u>Guided Review</u>

1. Describe the intoxication effects of cannabis.

2. What are some negative effects of cannabis use?

Club Drugs

<u>Guided Review</u>

1. What are some negative mental and physical health effects of ecstasy?

2. Describe the intoxication effects of the "date rape drugs," including GHB, ketamine, and rohypnol.

Theories of Substance Use, Abuse, and Dependence

<u>Key Term</u>

disease model:

<u>Guided Review</u>

1. Describe some of the ways that dopamine is influenced by substance use and how changes in dopamine neurons might produce dependence?

2. What is the evidence that genetics contribute to alcohol and substance dependence?

3. What is alcohol reactivity, and how might it contribute to drinking behavior?

4. How and why do men and women differ in terms of their sensitivity to alcohol?

5. Give some reasons why alcoholism should be viewed as a form of depression and some reasons why it should not.

6. Explain how modeling may contribute to patterns of alcohol use in families.

7. Explain how alcohol expectancies may contribute to drinking behavior.

8. What is behavioral undercontrol, and how is thought to influence substance use?

9. Give some reasons why the rates of alcohol use differ between men and women.

Treatment for Substance-Related Disorders

<u>Key Terms</u>

harm-reduction model:

detoxification:

antagonist drugs:

naltrexone:

naloxone:

disulfiram:

methadone:

methadone maintenance programs:

aversive classical conditioning:

covert sensitization therapy:

cue exposure and response prevention:

abstinence violation effect:

relapse prevention programs:

Guided Review

1. How do the disease model and harm-reduction approach differ?

2. Describe the appropriate use(s) of the following biological treatments: (1) benzodiazepines (2) antidepressants; (3) naltrexone; (4) naloxone; (5) disulfiram; and (6) methadone.

3. Describe how aversive classical conditioning, covert sensitization therapy, and cue exposure and response prevention work for the treatment of alcoholism.

4. Describe how cognitive techniques may be used to treat alcoholism.

5. What is the controlled drinking controversy? Describe the differing points of view on this topic.

6. What contributes to the abstinence violation effect?

7. Describe how relapse prevention programs may assist people to stop drinking.

8. What is Alcoholics Anonymous and how does it work?

9. Describe the Alcohol Skills Training Program (ASTP) and how it works.

10. Why might it be important to treat male and female substance abusers in different ways?

CASE EXAMPLE
Read the following description and answer the questions below:

Ben had a long history of violent and impulsive behavior, beginning when he was a preschooler, and continuing now that he is in his mid-twenties. He got into trouble constantly in school, and was eventually kicked out of high school for drinking on school property repeatedly. Ben has held a number of jobs for a short period of time. He has gotten fired from every one of these jobs because he came to work drunk or missed many days of work due to hangovers.

When Ben is drunk, he can get mean. He frequently picks fights with other men over trivial issues. He has hit his wife a number of times. Ben also will race off in his car when he is drunk, driving fast and erratically down the rural roads near where he lives. He has had a few accidents and lost his driver's license when he was caught driving drunk. He continues to drive without a license, however.

1. What substance-related disorder does Ben likely have? What symptoms of this disorder does he show?

2. What other Axis II disorder might Ben's symptoms indicate?

3. How would a cognitive-behavioral therapist treat Ben?

CHAPTER TEST

A. Multiple Choice. Choose the **best answer** to each question below.

1. Which of the following people would be diagnosed with a substance-related disorder?

    A. Someone who abuses alcohol but is not dependent on it.
    B. Someone who inhales antifreeze and experiences significant anxiety and hallucinations as a result.
    C. Someone who smokes rat poison and experiences mild, transient effects from it.
    D. Someone who uses opioids, but who does not exhibit significant tolerance or withdrawal symptoms.

2. Substance dependence is

    A. a diagnosis given when recurrent substance use leads to significant harmful consequences.
    B. the experience of clinically significant distress in social, occupational, or other areas of functioning due to the cessation or reduction of substance use.

C. the experience of significant maladaptive behavioral and psychological symptoms due to the effect of a substance on the central nervous system.
D. a diagnosis given when substance use leads to tolerance and withdrawal symptoms or significant impairment or distress.

3. A DSM-IV-TR diagnosis can be given for withdrawal symptoms from all of the following substances <u>except</u>:

    A. barbiturates.
    B. amphetamines.
    C. caffeine.
    D. nicotine.

4. Which of the following is <u>not</u> included in the diagnostic criteria for substance abuse?

    A. There is a persistent desire or unsuccessful efforts to cut down or control substance use.
    B. Failure to meet important obligations at work, school, or home.
    C. Use of the substance in situations in which it is physically hazardous to do so.
    D. Legal problems as a result of substance use.

5. Which of the following is <u>not</u> a criterion for substance dependence?

    A. The substance is often taken in larger amounts or over a longer period than was intended.
    B. Repeated legal problems as a result of substance use.
    C. A great deal of time is spent in activities necessary to obtain the substance, use the substance, or recover from its effects.
    D. Important social, occupational, or recreational activities are given up or reduced because of substance use.

6. All of the following are present among alcoholics with antisocial personalities more than in alcoholics without such personalities <u>except</u>

    A. more severe symptoms of alcoholism.
    B. heavier drug involvement.
    C. experience of depressive and anxiety symptoms as children.
    D. increased likelihood of coming from alcoholic families.

7. A loss of memory for recent events, problems in recalling distant events, and confabulation are features of

    A. Wernicke's encephalopathy.
    B. alcohol-induced dementia.
    C. substance intoxication.
    D. Korsakoff's psychosis.

8. The ethnic group at highest risk for alcohol abuse and dependence is

    A. Caucasians.
    B. African Americans.
    C. Native Americans.
    D. Hispanics.

9. Which of the following is a true explanation for why rates of alcohol problems are higher among older people?

    A. The rates of alcohol problems are actually lower, not higher, among older people.
    B. Older people have more free time and financial security than younger people, which makes it possible for them to tolerate hangovers and negative effects of alcohol.
    C. Older people have grown up under fewer prohibitions against alcohol use and abuse, since alcohol problems were much less common during their younger years.
    D. Older people metabolize alcohol at a slower rate than younger people, which leads them to become intoxicated more quickly.

10. Which of the following is a biological cause of cravings for a substance?

    A. Neural sensitization in the dopamine system
    B. Neural desensitization in the dopamine system
    C. Opponent processes
    D. Increased levels of serotonin

11. The sons of alcoholics have been found to exhibit all of the following characteristics except

    A. lower reactivity to moderate doses of alcohol.
    B. low physiological tolerance to alcohol, which leads them to achieve intoxication easily.
    C. high physiological tolerance to alcohol.
    D. significantly greater likelihood of becoming an alcoholic.

12. Which of the following statements about alcoholism and depression is true?

    A. Depression among alcoholics typically remains even after the alcoholism is treated.
    B. Alcohol-related disorders and depression run together in families.
    C. The odds of alcoholism preceding depression are lower than the odds of depression preceding alcoholism.
    D. Depressed adolescents are more likely to become alcoholics than those who are not depressed.

13. Alcohol cravings can be reduced with

    A. naloxone.

B. methadone.
C. disulfiram.
D. naltrexone.

14. A drug that makes the user feel sick and dizzy when he or she ingests alcohol is

    A. naloxone.
    B. methadone.
    C. disulfiram.
    D. naltrexone.

15. In which of the following treatments are alcoholics caused to experience their favorite types of alcohol, encouraged to hold glasses to their lips, and smell the alcohol, but are not allowed to drink any of the alcohol?

    A. Cue exposure and response prevention
    B. Aversive classical conditioning
    C. Covert sensitization therapy
    D. Controlled drinking treatment

16. The most widely-used illicit substance(s) in the world is/are

    A. inhalants.
    B. cannabis.
    C. cocaine.
    D. opioids.

17. Abuse of all of the following may be diagnosed in DSM-IV-TR except

    A. alcohol.
    B. nicotine.
    C. amphetamines.
    D. opioids.

18. Chronic use of _____ can result in eventual withdrawal symptoms of paranoia, memory loss, and mood instability that last weeks, months, and even years.

    A. alcohol
    B. caffeine
    C. amphetamines
    D. opioids

19. Delirium tremens can occur after withdrawal from

    A. alcohol.
    B. cocaine.

C. opioids.
D. hallucinogens.

20. The lowest rates of alcoholism are found in which of the following cultures?

    A. United States
    B. Germany
    C. Puerto Rico
    D. China

B. <u>True-False</u>. Select T (True) or F (False) below.

1. Women are less likely to quit smoking than men.   T   F

2. For a person to be diagnosed with substance dependence, he or she must exhibit both tolerance and withdrawal to the substance.   T   F

3. Binge drinking is no more common among members of fraternities and sororities than it is among the general college population.   T   F

4. Ecstasy users have significantly lower levels of serotonin than individuals who do not use ecstasy.   T   F

5. The use of cocaine has declined since the mid-1980s.   T   F

C. <u>Short Answer Questions</u>.

1. Give some examples of how substance use and abuse are regarded by different cultures.

2. How do the rates of alcohol disorders vary by culture, gender, and age? What are some of the proposed reasons for these differences?

3. Discuss the movement by the United States government to declare nicotine a drug, and provide arguments in favor of and against this idea.

4. Describe two cognitive-behavioral treatments and two biological treatments for alcoholism described in the chapter.

5. Contrast the disease model of alcoholism with the controlled drinking perspective. Do you think that some alcoholics can learn to control their drinking? Why or why not?

ANSWER KEY

<u>Case Example</u>
1. Alcohol dependence. He shows withdrawal symptoms (hangovers), continued use of alcohol despite several negative consequences (losing jobs, losing his license, being kicked out of school, getting into fights).
2. Antisocial personality disorder. He has a life-long history of violent and impulsive behavior that violates the fundamental rights of others (fights, hitting his wife, driving drunk and without a license).
3. First detoxification, perhaps using naltroxone to block the effects of the alcohol. Second, help him identify thoughts or situations that trigger impulsive behaviors and drinking. Third, help him develop alternative coping strategies for these situations and to challenge the thoughts that contribute to drinking.

<u>Multiple Choice</u>
1. B
2. D
3. C
4. A
5. B
6. C
7. D
8. C
9. A
10. A
11. B
12. B
13. D
14. C
15. A
16. B
17. B
18. C
19. A
20. D

<u>True-False</u>
1. T
2. F
3. F
4. T
5. T

Short Answer Questions
1. See pp. 621–623.
2. See pp. 634–636.
3. See pp. 643–645.
4. See pp. 660–663.
5. See pp. 663–664.

Additional Readings on Chapter 17 Topics
Babor, T. F., Aguirre-Molina, M., Marlatt, G. A., & Clayton, R. (1999). Managing alcohol problems and risky drinking. American Journal of Health Promotion, 14, 98-103.

Larimer, M. E., Palmer, R. S., & Marlatt, G. A. (1999). Relapse prevention: An overview of Marlatt's cognitive-behavioral model. Alcohol Research and Health, 23, 151-160.

Montoya, A. G., Sorrentino, R., Lukas, S. E., & Price, B. H. (2002). Long-term neuropsychiatric consequences of "Ecstasy" (MDMA): A review. Harvard Review of Psychiatry, 10, 212-220.

Chapter 18: Mental Health and the Law

LEARNING OBJECTIVES
After reading and studying this chapter, you should be able to:

1.   Discuss the limitations of psychological research to inform legal decisions.

2.   Discuss how competency to stand trial is determined.

3.   Discuss the characteristics of people most likely to be referred for competency evaluations, and the characteristics of people most likely to be found incompetent to stand trial.

4.   Discuss the frequency with which the insanity defense is used, and the typical judgments that result when it is used.

5.   Summarize how insanity pleas are evaluated according to the M'Naghten rule, irresistible impulse rule, Durham rule, ALI rule, and the American Psychiatric Association's definition of insanity.

6.   Discuss the pros and cons of each rule above and describe how each rule either broadened or constricted the legal definition of insanity.

7.   Discuss the significance of *Barrett v. United States* (1977).

8.   Discuss the use of the guilty but mentally ill (GBMI) verdict.

9.   Discuss the need for treatment as a justification for civil commitment.

10.   Discuss the modern criteria used to enable civil commitment, and the variations in how states treat the legal issue of civil commitment.

11.   Discuss the significance of *Donaldson v. O'Connor* (1975).

12.   Describe the factors that predict violence over the short term.

13.   Describe the prevalence of violence among mentally ill people.

14.   Describe the prevalence of involuntary commitment.

15.   Discuss the rights of patients to receive treatment and to refuse treatment.

16.   Discuss the circumstances in which patients' rights can be violated.

17.   Identify and describe the clinician's duties to the client and society.

18.   Discuss when confidentiality may be broken, and when it may not be broken.

ESSENTIAL IDEAS

I. Judgments about people accused of crimes

    A. One judgment mental-health professionals are asked to make is about an accused person's competence to stand trial.

    B. Another judgment is whether the accused person was "sane" at the time he or she committed a crime.

    C. The insanity defense has undergone many changes over recent history, often in response to its use in high profile crimes.

    D. Five rules have been used to evaluate the acceptability of a plea of not guilty by reason of insanity: the M'Naghten rule, the irresistible impulse rule, the Durham rule, the ALI rule, and the American Psychiatric Association definition of insanity.

    E. All of these rules require that the defendant be diagnosed with a "mental disease" but do not clearly define *mental disease*.

    F. Most of these rules also require that the defendant is unable to understand the criminality of his or her actions or conform his or her actions to the law in order to be judged not guilty by reason of insanity.

    G. Many states have introduced the alternative verdict of guilty but mentally ill.

II. Involuntary commitment and civil rights

    A. People can be held in mental health facilities involuntarily if they are judged to have grave disabilities that make it difficult for them to meet their own basic needs or that pose imminent danger to themselves or to others. Each of the criteria used to make such judgments has its flaws, however, creating concerns about the appropriateness of civil commitment.

    B. Short-term commitments can occur without court hearings based on the certification of mental health professionals that individuals are in emergency situations. Such commitments are most likely to happen for individuals who are actively suicidal.

    C. Longer-term commitments require court hearings. Patients have the rights to have an attorney and to appeal rulings.

    D. Other basic rights of patients are the right to be treated while being hospitalized and the right to refuse treatment (at least in some states).

E. Research shows higher rates of violence by people with mental disorders, particularly those who also have a history of substance abuse, but the rates are not as high as some stereotypes would suggest.

III. Clinicians' duties to clients and society

A. First and foremost, clinicians have a duty to provide competent care to their clients.

B. Clinicians must also avoid multiple relationships with their clients, particularly sexual relationships.

C. They must protect their clients' confidentiality, except under special circumstances. One of these special circumstances occurs when a therapist believes a client needs to be committed involuntarily.

D. Two other duties therapists have to society—the duty to protect people clients are threatening to harm, and the duty to report suspected child or elder abuse—require them to break clients' confidentiality.

E. Recently, clinicians have been charged with providing ethical service to diverse populations.

KEY TERMS AND GUIDED REVIEW

Key Term

mentally ill:

Guided Review

1. What are some limitations on the ability of mental health professionals to assist the law and society?

Judgments About People Accused of Crimes

Key Terms

incompetent to stand trial:

insanity:

insanity defense:

M'Naghten rule:

irresistible impulse rule:

Durham rule:

ALI rule:

Insanity Defense Reform Act:

American Psychiatric Association definition of insanity:

guilty but mentally ill (GBMI):

Guided Review

1. Give some examples of impairments that might lead an individual to be regarded as incompetent to stand trial.

2. What are some characteristics of people that increase their likelihood of being considered incompetent to stand trial?

3. What is the fundamental premise underlying the insanity defense?

4. How often do people plead not guilty by reason of insanity, and how often is this plea successful?

5. What happens to defendants who are found not guilty by reason of insanity?

6. What is the M'Naghten Rule? What are two major problems with it?

7. How did the irresistible impulse rule broaden the legal definition of insanity over the M'Naghten rule?

8. What was the Durham Rule, and what was its major flaw?

9. What is the ALI Rule? Explain how it is broader than the M'Naghten Rule but not as broad as the Durham Rule.

10. What was the significance of *Barrett v. United States* (1977)?

11. What is the American Psychiatric Association definition of insanity?

12. What are some arguments for and against the GBMI verdict?

Involuntary Commitment and Civil Rights

Key Terms

need for treatment:

civil commitment:

grave disability:

dangerousness to self:

dangerousness to others:

right to treatment:

right to refuse treatment:

informed consent:

<u>Guided Review</u>

1. Describe some of the problems with the "need for treatment" criterion for civil commitment.

2. What are the current criteria used to determine if someone should be committed involuntarily?

3. What is the significance of *Donaldson v. O'Connor* (1975)?

4. Which patients are most likely to engage in violence after being discharged, and who are their most common targets?

5. How common are involuntary admissions to psychiatric hospitals?

6. What is the significance of *Wyatt v. Stickney* (1972)?

7. How common are mental disorders among prison inmates? How do the diagnoses vary by gender?

8. What are some limitations of the right to refuse treatment?

Clinicians' Duties to Clients and Society

<u>Guided Review</u>

1. Why do clinicians have a duty not to become involved in multiple relationships with clients?

2. How often do clinicians have sexual relationships with their clients?

3. What is the significance of *Tarasoff v. Regents of the University of California* (1974)?

4. What are the conditions under which a clinician may appropriately violate a client's confidentiality?

CHAPTER TEST

A. <u>Multiple Choice</u>. Choose the **best answer** to each question below.

1. All of the following increase one's likelihood of being judged incompetent to stand trial <u>except</u>:

    A. being female.
    B. being Caucasian.
    C. being poorly educated.
    D. being accused of a violent crime.

2. The insanity defense

    A. will only be successful if it can be proven that the defendant has been chronically insane.
    B. is usually successful when it is used as one's plea.
    C. is most often used to acquit individuals with schizophrenia.
    D. is used in only about 5 percent of felony cases.

3. The idea that someone cannot be held responsible for a crime if he did not know the nature or quality of the act being performed, or if he did not know that his actions were wrong, is known as the

    A. M'Naghten rule.
    B. Durham rule.
    C. ALI rule.
    D. irresistible impulse rule.

4. The condition most commonly recognized as a "disease of the mind" is

    A. severe depression.
    B. psychosis.
    C. alcoholism.
    D. antisocial personality disorder.

5. A person can still be found not guilty by reason of insanity even if she knows the act she performed is wrong (i.e., criminal) under which of the following legal principles?

    A. The ALI rule
    B. The M'Naghten rule

C. The American Psychiatric Association definition of insanity

D. The Durham rule

6. The case that established that the voluntary use of alcohol and drugs does not qualify as a "mental disease or defect" for the purposes of determining insanity was

    A. *Durham v. United States* (1954).

    B. *Donaldson v. O' Connor* (1975).

    C. *Wyatt v. Stickney* (1972).

    D. *Barrett v. United States* (1977).

7. The Insanity Defense Reform Act adopted which of the following legal definitions of insanity?

    A. The ALI rule

    B. The M'Naghten rule

    C. The American Psychiatric Association definition of insanity

    D. The irresistible impulse rule

8. If an individual is not held responsible for a crime because, at the time of the crime, as a result of mental disease or defect, the person lacked substantial capacity either to appreciate the criminality (wrongfulness) of the act or to conform his behavior to the law, the ruling uses which of the following criteria?

    A. The ALI rule

    B. The M'Naghten rule

    C. The American Psychiatric Association definition of insanity

    D. The Durham rule

9. An argument against the guilty but mentally ill (GBMI) verdict is

    A. that it allows defendants to return home rather than face incarceration.

    B. that it does not hold defendants responsible for their actions.

    C. that it does not adequately recognize the mental illness of defendants.

    D. that there is no guarantee that the defendant will receive treatment.

10. Which of the following is <u>not</u> a criterion used to commit someone to a psychiatric facility?

    A. Imminent danger to self

    B. Imminent danger to others

    C. Diagnosis of a mental disorder

    D. Need for treatment

11. *Donaldson v. O'Connor* (1975) established

    A. the right to treatment.

B. the unconstitutionality of confining a non-dangerous individual.
C. the clinician's duty to protect others from harm.
D. the need to refine the irresistible impulse rule.

12. Which of the following is one of the best predictors of violence over a short term?

A. Having a diagnosis of schizophrenia
B. Being male
C. Having a diagnosis of substance abuse
D. Being Caucasian

13. Violence among people who have been discharged from a psychiatric hospital

A. most often targets strangers.
B. occurs more frequently among mentally ill men.
C. occurs more frequently among mentally ill African Americans.
D. does not occur among the majority of people.

14. *Wyatt v. Stickney* (1972) established

A. the right to treatment.
B. the unconstitutionality of confining a non-dangerous individual.
C. the duty of clinicians to protect patient confidentiality.
D. the right to refuse treatment.

15. Studies of female prison inmates have shown that the most common mental disorder in that population is

A. antisocial personality disorder.
B. substance abuse or dependence.
C. major depression.
D. borderline personality disorder.

16. Which of the following cases established the clinician's duty to protect people who might be in danger because of his or her client?

A. *Durham v. United States* (1954)
B. *Tarasoff v. Regents of The University of California* (1974)
C. *Donaldson v. O' Connor* (1975)
D. *Wyatt v. Stickney* (1972)

17. The right to refuse treatment

A. is a basic right adopted by all states and the federal system.
B. cannot be contested by family members or treating clinicians.
C. is not recognized in some states.

D. is reserved for patients with severe psychotic disorders.

18. Which of the following is <u>not</u> a guideline for ethical service to culturally diverse populations?

    A. Psychologists avoid racist practices and do not consider ethnicity or culture as significant parameters in understanding psychological processes; rather, they emphasize the individual client.
    B. Psychologists are cognizant of relevant research and practice issues as related to the population being served.
    C. Psychologists interact in the language requested by the client and, if this is not feasible, make an appropriate referral.
    D. Psychologists attend to, as well as work to eliminate, biases, prejudices, and discriminatory practices.

19. Clinicians may <u>not</u> violate a client's confidentiality

    A. to report suspected child abuse.
    B. to report suspected abuse of elderly persons.
    C. to consult with the client's physician about his or her symptoms.
    D. to protect persons who might be in danger because of their client.

20. A sexual relationship between a therapist and a client

    A. is a felony in some states.
    B. is frowned upon but is not considered unethical or illegal.
    C. is not considered unethical if the client consents to the relationship.
    D. is not considered unethical if the relationship occurs at least 6 months after the therapeutic relationship has ended.

B. <u>True-False</u>. Select T (True) or F (False) below.

1. Insanity is a legal term, not a psychological term.   T   F

2. Women are more likely to be acquitted by reason of insanity than are men.   T   F

3. Mentally ill men are more likely to be violent than are mentally ill women.   T   F

4. A requirement for competence to stand trial is that the defendant has no history of mental illness.   T   F

5. Prison inmates have a right to mental health treatment.   T   F

C. <u>Short Answer Questions</u>.

1. Which types of people are most likely to be acquitted by reason of insanity? How common are such acquittals?

2. What is the American Psychiatric Association's definition of insanity? How is it similar to and different from the M'Naghten rule and ALI rule?

3. What are the criteria used to commit someone to a psychiatric facility involuntarily? Explain each of these criteria.

4. Why do clinicians have a duty to protect clients' confidentiality? Under what circumstances might a clinician justifiably violate a client's confidentiality? Give two examples of when a clinician should not violate a client's confidentiality.

5. Discuss the relationship between mental illness and violence, and indicate which mentally ill patients are most likely to become violent.

ANSWER KEY

<u>Multiple Choice</u>
1. B
2. C
3. A
4. B
5. D
6. D
7. C
8. A
9. D
10. D
11. B
12. C
13. D
14. A
15. B
16. B
17. C
18. A
19. C
20. A

<u>True-False</u>
1. T
2. F
3. F
4. F
5. T

<u>Short Answer Questions</u>
1. See p. 680.
2. See pp. 682–684.
3. See pp. 685–687.
4. See p. 692.
5. See pp. 687–689.

Additional Readings on Chapter 18 Topics

Alper, J. S. (1998). Genes, free will and criminal responsibility. *Social Science and Medicine, 46,* 1599-1611.

Berman, M. E., & Coccaro, E. F. (1998). Neurobiologic correlates of violence: Relevance to criminal responsibility. *Behavioral Sciences and the Law, 16,* 303-318.

Grisso, T., Steinberg, L., Woolard, J., Cauffman, E., Scott, E., Graham, S., Lexcen, F., Reppucci, N. D., & Schwartz, R. (2003). Juveniles' competence to stand trial: A comparison of adolescents' and adults' capacities as trial defendants. *Law and Human Behavior, 27,* 333-363.